STATISTICS WITH CONFIDENCE

D0862710

*This book is dedicated to the memory of
Martin and Linda Gardner.*

STATISTICS WITH CONFIDENCE

Confidence intervals and statistical guidelines

Second edition

Edited by

DOUGLAS G ALTMAN
Director, Imperial Cancer Research Fund Medical Statistics Group and Centre for Statistics in Medicine, Oxford

DAVID MACHIN
Director, National Medical Research Council, Clinical Trials and Epidemiology Research Unit, Singapore

TREVOR N BRYANT
Senior Lecturer in Biocomputation, University of Southampton

and

MARTIN J GARDNER
Former Professor of Medical Statistics, MRC Environmental Epidemiology Unit, University of Southampton

First published 1989
Reprinted 1989
Reprinted 1990 (3 times)
Reprinted 1992
Reprinted 1993
Reprinted 1994
Reprinted 1995
Reprinted 1996
Reprinted 1998
Second edition 2000

British Library Cataloguing in Publication Data
A catalogue record for this book is available from the British Library.

ISBN 0 7279 1375 1

Typeset by Academic + Technical Typesetting, Bristol
Printed by J W Arrowsmith Ltd, Bristol

Contents

v

PART II   STATISTICAL GUIDELINES AND CHECKLISTS

PART III   NOTATION, SOFTWARE, AND TABLES

Contributors

Douglas G Altman, *Director, Imperial Cancer Research Fund Medical Statistics Group and Centre for Statistics in Medicine, Institute of Health Sciences, Oxford*

Trevor N Bryant, *Senior Lecturer in Biocomputation, Medical Statistics and Computing (University of Southampton), Southampton General Hospital, Southampton*

Michael J Campbell, *Professor of Medical Statistics, Institute of Primary Care, University of Sheffield, Northern General Hospital, Sheffield*

Leslie E Daly, *Associate Professor of Public Health Medicine and Epidemiology, University College Dublin, Ireland*

Martin J Gardner, *former Professor of Medical Statistics, MRC Environmental Epidemiology Unit (University of Southampton), Southampton General Hospital, Southampton*

Sheila M Gore, *Senior Medical Statistician, MRC Biostatistics Unit, Cambridge*

David Machin,⋆ *Director, National Medical Research Council Clinical Trials and Epidemiology Research Unit, Ministry of Health, Singapore*

Julie A Morris, *Medical Statistician, Department of Medical Statistics, Withington Hospital, West Didsbury, Manchester*

Robert G Newcombe, *Senior Lecturer in Medical Statistics, University of Wales College of Medicine, Cardiff*

Stuart J Pocock, *Professsor of Medical Statistics, London School of Hygiene and Tropical Medicine, London*

⋆ Now *Professor of Clinical Trials Research, University of Sheffield*

Source of contents

15   Gardner MJ, Machin D, Campbell MJ. Use of checklists in assessing the statistical content of medical studies. *BMJ* 1986;**292**:810–2 (revised and expanded)

PART III   Notation, software and tables

Introduction

DOUGLAS G ALTMAN, DAVID MACHIN,
TREVOR N BRYANT

In preparing a new edition of a book, the editors are usually happy in the knowledge that the first edition has been a success. In the current circumstances, this satisfaction is tinged with deep personal regret that Martin Gardner, the originator of the idea for *Statistics with Confidence*, died in 1993 aged just 52. His achievements in a prematurely shortened career were outlined in his obituary in the *BMJ*.[1]

The first edition of *Statistics with Confidence* (1989) was essentially a collection of expository articles concerned with confidence intervals and statistical guidelines that had been published in the *BMJ* over the period 1986 to 1988. All were co-authored by Martin. The other contributors were Douglas Altman, Michael Campbell, Sheila Gore, David Machin, Julie Morris and Stuart Pocock. The whole book was translated into Italian[2] and the statistical guidelines have also appeared in Spanish.[3]

As may be expected, several developments have occurred since the publication of the first edition and Martin had discussed and agreed some of the changes that we have now introduced into this new and expanded edition. Notably, this second edition includes new chapters on Diagnostic tests (chapter 10); Clinical trials and meta-analyses (chapter 11); Confidence intervals and sample sizes (chapter 12); and Special topics (substitution method, exact and mid-P confidence intervals, bootstrap confidence intervals, and multiple comparisons) (chapter 13). There is also a review of the impact of confidence intervals in the medical literature over the ten years or so since the first edition (chapter 2). All the chapters from the first edition have been revised, some extensively, and one (chapter 6 on proportions) has been completely rewritten. The list of contributors has been extended to include Leslie Daly and Robert Newcombe. We are grateful to readers of the first edition for constructive comments which have assisted us in preparing this revision.

Alongside the first edition of *Statistics with Confidence*, a computer program, Confidence Interval Analysis (CIA), was available. This program, which could carry out the calculations described in the book, had been written by Martin, his son Stephen Gardner and Paul Winter. An entirely new Windows version of CIA has been written by Trevor Bryant to accompany the book, and is packaged with this second edition. It is outlined in chapter 17. The program reflects the changes made for this edition of the book and has been influenced by suggestions from users.

Despite the enhanced coverage we would reiterate the comment in the introduction to the first edition, that this book is not intended as a comprehensive statistical textbook. For further details of statistical methods the reader is referred to other sources.[4-7]

We were all privileged to be colleagues of Martin Gardner. We hope that he would have approved of this new edition of *Statistics with Confidence* and would be pleased to know that he is still associated with it. In 1995 the Royal Statistical Society posthumously awarded Martin the inaugural Bradford Hill medal for his important contributions to medical statistics. The medal was accepted by his widow Linda. As we were completing this second edition in October 1999 we were greatly saddened to learn that Linda too had died from cancer, far too young. We dedicate this book to the memory of both Martin and Linda Gardner.

1 Obituary of MJ Gardner. *BMJ* 1993;**306**:387.
2 Gardner MJ, Altman DG (eds) *Gli intervalli di confidenza. Oltre la significatività statistica*. Rome: Il Pensiero Scientifico Editore, 1990.
3 Altman DG, Gore SM, Gardner MJ, Pocock SJ. Normas estadisticas para los colaboradores de revistas de medicina. *Archivos de Bronconeumologia* 1988; **24**:48–56.
4 Altman DG. *Practical statistics for medical research*. London: Chapman & Hall, 1991.
5 Armitage P, Berry G. *Statistical methods in medical research*. 3rd edn. Oxford: Blackwell Science, 1994.
6 Bland M. *An introduction to medical statistics*. 3rd edn. Oxford: Oxford University Press, 2000.
7 Campbell MJ, Machin D. *Medical statistics. A commonsense approach*. 3rd edn. Chichester: John Wiley, 1999.

Part I
Estimation and confidence intervals

1 Estimating with confidence

MARTIN J GARDNER, DOUGLAS G ALTMAN

Editors' note: this chapter is reproduced from the first edition (with minor adjustments). It was closely based on an editorial published in 1988 in the British Medical Journal. *Chapter 2 describes developments in the use of confidence intervals in the medical literature since 1988.*

Statistical analysis of medical studies is based on the key idea that we make observations on a sample of subjects and then draw inferences about the population of all such subjects from which the sample is drawn. If the study sample is not representative of the population we may well be misled and statistical procedures cannot help. But even a well-designed study can give only an idea of the answer sought because of random variation in the sample. Thus results from a single sample are subject to statistical uncertainty, which is strongly related to the size of the sample. Examples of the statistical analysis of sample data would be calculating the difference between the proportions of patients improving on two treatment regimens or the slope of the regression line relating two variables. These quantities will be imprecise estimates of the values in the overall population, but fortunately the imprecision can itself be estimated and incorporated into the presentation of findings. Presenting study findings directly on the scale of original measurement, together with information on the inherent imprecision due to sampling variability, has distinct advantages over just giving P values usually dichotomised into "significant" or "non-significant". This is the rationale for using confidence intervals.

The main purpose of confidence intervals is to indicate the (im)precision of the sample study estimates as population values. Consider the following points for example: a difference of 20% between the percentages improving in two groups of 80 patients having treatments A and B was reported, with a 95% confidence interval of 6% to 34% (see chapter 5). Firstly, a possible difference in treatment effectiveness of less than 6% or of more than 34% is not excluded by such values being outside the confidence interval—they are simply less likely than those inside the confidence interval. Secondly, the middle half of the 95% confidence interval (from 13% to 27%) is more likely to contain the population value than the extreme two quarters (6% to 13% and 27% to 34%)—in fact the middle half forms a 67% confidence interval. Thirdly, regardless of the width of the confidence interval, the sample estimate is the best indicator of the population value—in this case a 20% difference in treatment response.

The *British Medical Journal* now expects scientific papers submitted to it to contain confidence intervals when appropriate.[1] It also wants a reduced emphasis on the presentation of P values from hypothesis testing (see chapter 3). *The Lancet,*[2,3] the *Medical Journal of Australia,*[4] the *American Journal of Public Health,*[5] and the *British Heart Journal,*[6] have implemented the same policy, and it has been endorsed by the International Committee of Medical Journal Editors.[7] One of the blocks to implementing the policy had been that the methods needed to calculate confidence intervals are not readily available in most statistical textbooks. The chapters that follow present appropriate techniques for most common situations. Further articles in the *American Journal of Public Health* and the *Annals of Internal Medicine* have debated the uses of confidence intervals and hypothesis tests and discussed the interpretation of confidence intervals.[8-14]

So when should confidence intervals be calculated and presented? Essentially confidence intervals become relevant whenever an inference is to be made from the study results to the wider world. Such an inference will relate to summary, not individual, characteristics—for example, rates, differences in medians, regression coefficients, etc. The calculated interval will give us a range of values within which we can have a chosen confidence of it containing the population value. The most usual degree of confidence presented is 95%, but any suggestion to standardise on 95%[2,3] would not seem desirable.[15]

Thus, a single study usually gives an imprecise sample estimate of the overall population value in which we are interested. This imprecision is indicated by the width of the confidence interval: the wider the interval the less the precision. The width depends essentially on three factors. Firstly, the sample size: larger sample sizes will give more precise results with narrower confidence intervals (see chapter 3). In particular, wide confidence intervals emphasise the unreliability of conclusions based on small samples. Secondly, the variability of the characteristic being studied: the less variable it is (between subjects, within subjects, from measurement error, and from other sources) the more precise the sample estimate and the narrower the confidence interval. Thirdly, the degree of confidence required: the more confidence the wider the interval.

1 Langman MJS. Towards estimation and confidence intervals. *BMJ* 1986;**292**:716.
2 Anonymous. Report with confidence [Editorial]. *Lancet* 1987;**i**:488.
3 Bulpitt CJ. Confidence intervals. *Lancet* 1987;**i**:494–7.
4 Berry G. Statistical significance and confidence intervals. *Med J Aust* 1986;**144**:618–19
5 Rothman KJ, Yankauer A. Confidence intervals vs significance tests: quantitative interpretation (Editors' note). *Am J Public Health* 1986;**76**:587–8.
6 Evans SJW, Mills P, Dawson J. The end of the P value? *Br Heart J* 1988;**60**:177–80.
7 International Committee of Medical Journal Editors. Uniform requirements for manuscripts submitted to biomedical journals. *BMJ* 1988;**296**:401–5.
8 DeRouen TA, Lachenbruch PA, Clark VA, *et al*. Four comments received on statistical testing and confidence intervals. *Am J Public Health* 1987;**77**:237–8.
9 Anonymous. Four comments received on statistical testing and confidence intervals. *Am J Public Health* 1987;**77**:238.
10 Thompson WD. Statistical criteria in the interpretation of epidemiological data. *Am J Public Health* 1987;**77**:191–4.
11 Thompson WD. On the comparison of effects. *Am J Public Health* 1987;**77**:491–2.
12 Poole C. Beyond the confidence interval. *Am J Public Health* 1987;**77**:195–9.
13 Poole C. Confidence intervals exclude nothing. *Am J Public Health* 1987;**77**:492–3.
14 Braitman, LE. Confidence intervals extract clinically useful information from data. *Ann Intern Med* 1988;**108**:296–8.
15 Gardner MJ, Altman DG. Using confidence intervals. *Lancet* 1987;**i**:746.

2 Confidence intervals in practice

DOUGLAS G ALTMAN

As noted in chapter 1, confidence intervals are not a modern device, yet their use in medicine (and indeed other scientific areas) was quite unusual until the second half of the 1980s. For some reason in the mid-1980s there was a spate of interest in the topic, with many journals publishing editorials and expository articles (see chapter 1). It seems that several such articles in leading medical journals were particularly influential. Since the first edition of this book there have been many further such publications, often contrasting confidence intervals and significance tests. There has been a continuing increase in the use of confidence intervals in medical research papers, although some medical specialties seem somewhat slower to move in this direction. This chapter briefly summarises some of this literature.

Surveys of the use of confidence intervals in medical journals

There is a long tradition of reviewing the statistical content of medical journals, and several recent reviews have included the use of confidence intervals. Of particular interest is a review of the use of statistics in papers in the *British Medical Journal* in 1977 and 1994, before and after it adopted its policy of requiring authors to use confidence intervals.[1] One of the most marked increases was in the use of confidence intervals, which had risen from 4% to 62% of papers using some statistical technique, a large increase but still well short of that required. Similarly, between 1980 and 1990 the use of confidence intervals in the *American Journal of Epidemiology* approximately doubled to 70%, and it was around 90% in the subset of papers related to cancer,[2] despite a lack of editorial directive.[3] This review also illustrated a wider phenomenon, that the increased use of confidence intervals was not so much instead of P values but as a supplement to them.[2]

The uptake of confidence intervals has not been equal throughout medicine. A review of papers published in the *American Journal of Physiology* in 1996 found that out of 370 papers only one reported confidence intervals![4] They were presented in just 16% of 100 papers in two radiology journals in 1993 compared with 52% of 50 concurrent papers in the *British Medical Journal*.[5]

Confidence intervals may also be uncommon in certain contexts. For example, they were used in only 2 of 112 articles in anaesthesia journals (in 1991–92) in conjunction with analyses of data from visual analogue scales.[6]

Editorials and expository articles

Editorials[7–19] and expository articles[20–31] related to confidence intervals have continued to appear in medical journals, some being quite lengthy and detailed. In effect, the authors have almost all favoured greater use of confidence intervals and reduced use of P values (a few exceptions are discussed below). Many of these papers have contrasted estimation and confidence intervals with significance tests and P values.

Such articles seem to have become rarer in the second half of the 1990s, which may indicate that confidence intervals are now routinely included in introductory statistics courses, that there is a wide belief that this particular battle has been won, or that their use is so widespread that researchers use them to conform. Probably all of these are true to some degree.

Medical journal policy

As noted in chapter 1, when the first edition of this book was published in 1989, a few medical journals had begun to include some mention of confidence intervals in their instructions to authors. In 1988 the influential 'Vancouver guidelines'[32] (originally published in 1979) included the following passage:

> Describe statistical methods with enough detail to enable a knowledgeable reader with access to the original data to verify the reported results. When possible, quantify findings and present them with appropriate indicators of measurement error or uncertainty (such as confidence intervals). Avoid relying solely on statistical hypothesis

7

testing, such as the use of P values, which fails to convey important quantitative information.

This passage has survived intact to May 1999 apart from one trivial rewording.[33] The comment on confidence intervals is, however, very brief and rather nebulous. In 1988 Bailar and Mosteller published a helpful amplification of the Vancouver section,[34] but this article is not cited in recent versions of the guidelines. Over 500 medical journals have agreed to use the Vancouver requirements in their instructions to authors.[33]

Despite the continuing flow of editorials in medical journals in favour of greater use of confidence intervals,[7–19] it is clear that the uptake of this advice has been patchy, as illustrated by reviews of published papers and also journals' instructions to authors. In 1993, I reviewed the 'Instructions to Authors' of 135 journals, chosen to have high impact factors within their specialties. Only 19 (14%) mentioned confidence intervals explicitly in their instructions for authors, although about half made some mention of the Vancouver guidelines. Journals' instructions to authors change frequently, and not necessarily in the anticipated direction. Statistical guidelines published (anonymously) in 1993 in *Diabetic Medicine* included the following: 'Confidence intervals should be used to indicate the precision of estimated effects and differences'.[35] At the same time they published an editorial stating '*Diabetic Medicine* is now requesting the use of confidence intervals wherever possible'.[14] These two publications are not referenced in the 1999 guidelines, however, and there is no explicit mention of confidence intervals, although there is a reference to the Vancouver guidelines.[36]

Kenneth Rothman was an early advocate of confidence intervals in medical papers.[37] In 1986 he wrote: 'Testing for significance continues today not on its merits as a methodological tool but on the momentum of tradition. Rather than serving as a thinker's tool, it has become for some a clumsy substitute for thought, subverting what should be a contemplative exercise into an algorithm prone to error.'[38] Subsequently, as editor of *Epidemiology*, he has gone further:[39]

When writing for *Epidemiology*, you can also enhance your prospects if you omit tests of statistical significance. Despite a widespread belief that many journals require significance tests for publication, the Uniform Requirements for Manuscripts Submitted to Biomedical Journals discourages them, and every worthwhile journal will accept papers that omit them entirely. In *Epidemiology*, we do not publish them at all. Not only do we eschew publishing claims of the presence or absence of statistical significance, we discourage the use of this type of thinking in the data analysis, such as in the use of stepwise regression.

Curiously, this information is not given in the journal's 'Guidelines for Contributors' (http://www.epidem.com/), perhaps reflecting the slightly softer position of a 1997 editorial: 'it would be too dogmatic simply to ban the reporting of all P-values from *Epidemiology*.'[40] Despite widespread encouragement to include confidence intervals, I am unaware of any other medical journal which has taken such a strong stance against P values.

A relevant issue is the inclusion of confidence intervals in abstracts of papers. Many commentators have noted that the abstract is the most read part of a paper,[41] yet it is clear that it is the part that receives the least attention by authors, and perhaps also by editors. A few journals explicitly state in their instructions that abstracts should include confidence intervals. However, confidence intervals are often not included in the abstracts of papers even in journals which have signed up to guidelines requiring such presentation.[42,43]

Misuse of confidence intervals

The most obvious example of the misuse of confidence intervals is the presentation in a comparative study of separate confidence intervals for each group rather than a confidence interval for the contrast, as is recommended (chapter 14). This practice leads to inferences based on whether the two separate confidence intervals, such as for the means in each group, overlap or not. This is not the appropriate comparison and may mislead (see chapters 3 and 11). Of 100 consecutive papers (excluding randomised trials) that I refereed for the *British Medical Journal*, 8 papers out of the 59 (14%) which used confidence intervals used them inappropriately.[44]

The use for small samples of statistical methods intended for large samples can cause problems. In particular, confidence intervals for quantities constrained between limits should not include values outside the range of possible values for the quantities concerned. For example, the confidence interval for a proportion should not go outside the range 0 to 1 (or 0% to 100%) (see chapters 6 and 10). Quoted confidence intervals which include impossible values – such as the sensitivity of a diagnostic test greater than 100%, the area under the ROC curve greater than 1, and negative values of the odds ratio – should not be accepted by journals.[45,46]

One criticism of confidence intervals as used is that many researchers seem concerned only with whether the confidence interval includes the 'null' value representing no difference between the groups. Confidence intervals wholly to one side of the no effect point are deemed to indicate a significant result. This practice, which is based on a correct link between confidence interval and the P value, is indeed common. But even if the author of a paper acts in this way, by presenting the confidence interval they give readers the opportunity to take a different and more informative interpretation. When results are presented simply as P values, this option is unavailable.

Dissenting voices

It is clear that there is a considerable consensus among statisticians that confidence intervals represent a far better approach to the presentation and interpretation of results than significance tests and P values. Apart from those, mostly statisticians, who criticise all frequentist approaches to statistical inference (usually in favour of Bayesian methods), there seem to have been very few who have spoken out against the general view that confidence intervals are a much better way to present results than P values.

In a short editorial in the *Journal of Obstetrics and Gynecology*, the editor attacked several targets including confidence intervals.[47] He expressed the unshakeable view that only positive results (P < 0.05) indicate important findings, and suggested that 'The adoption of the [confidence interval] approach has already enabled the publication in full of many large but inconclusive studies...' Charlton[48] argued that confidence intervals do not provide information of any value to clinicians. In fact, he criticised confidence intervals for not doing something which they do not purport to do, namely indicate the variation in response for individual patients.

Hilden[49] cautioned that confidence intervals should not be presented 'when there are major threats to accuracy besides sampling error; or when a characteristic is too local and study-dependent to be generalizable'. Hall[50] took this line of reasoning further, arguing that confidence intervals 'should be used sparingly, if at all' when presenting the results of clinical trials. He also argued, contrary to the common view, that they might be particularly misleading 'when a clinical trial has failed to produce anticipated results'. His reasoning was that patients in a trial are not a random sample and thus the results cannot be generalised, and also that 'a clinical trial is designed to confirm expectation of treatment efficacy by rejecting the null hypothesis that differences are due to chance'. He went further, and suggested that 'there are few, if any, situations in which a confidence interval proves useful'. This line of reasoning has a rational basis, but he has taken it to unreasonable extremes. Other articles in the same journal issue[51,52] presented a more mainstream view.

It is interesting that there is no consensus among this small group of critics about what are the failings of confidence intervals. It is right to observe that we should always think carefully about the appropriate use and interpretation of *all* statistics, but it is wrong to suggest that all confidence intervals are meaningless or misleading.

Comment

Like many innovations, it is hard now to imagine the medical literature without confidence intervals. Overall, this is surely a development of great value, not least for the associated down-playing (but by no means elimination) of the wide use of $P < 0.05$ or $P > 0.05$ as a rule for interpreting study findings. However, as noted, confidence intervals can be both misused and overused and there are arguments in favour of other approaches to statistical inference. Also, despite a large increase in the use of confidence intervals, even in those journals which require confidence intervals – such as the *British Medical Journal* – their use is not widespread, and in some fields, such as physiology and psychology, their use remains uncommon.

Confidence intervals are especially valuable to aid the interpretation of clinical trials and meta-analyses[53] (see chapter 11). In cases where the estimated treatment effect is small the confidence interval indicates where clinically valuable treatment benefit remains plausible in the light of the data, and may help to avoid mistaking lack of evidence of effectiveness with evidence of lack of effectiveness.[54] The CONSORT statement[43] for reporting randomised trials requires confidence intervals, as does the QUOROM statement[55] for reporting systematic reviews and meta-analyses (see chapters 11 and 15).

11

None of this is meant to imply that confidence intervals offer a cure for all the problems associated with significance testing and P values, as several observers have noted.[56,57] We should certainly expect continuing developments in thinking about statistical inference.[58-61]

1 Seldrup J. Whatever happened to the *t*-test? *Drug Inf J* 1997;**31**:745–50.
2 Savitz DA, Tolo K-A, Poole C. Statistical significance testing in the *American Journal of Epidemiology*, 1970–1990. *Am J Epidemiol* 1994;**139**:1047–52.
3 Walter SD. Methods of reporting statistical results from medical research studies. *Am J Epidemiol* 1995;**141**:896–908.
4 Curran-Everett D, Taylor S, Kafadar K. Fundamental concepts in statistics: elucidation and illustration. *J Appl Physiol* 1998;**85**:775–86.
5 Cozens NJA. Should we have confidence intervals in radiology papers? *Clin Radiol* 1994;**49**:199–201.
6 Mantha S, Thisted R, Foss J, Ellis JE, Roizen MF. A proposal to use confidence intervals for visual analog scale data for pain measurement to determine clinical significance. *Anesth Analg* 1993;**77**:1041–7.
7 Keiding N. Sikkerhedsintervaller. *Ugeskr Læger* 1990;**152**:2622.
8 Braitman LE. Confidence intervals assess both clinical significance and statistical significance. *Ann Intern Med* 1991;**114**:515–17.
9 Russell I. Statistics – with confidence? *Br J Gen Pract* 1991;**41**:179–80.
10 Altman DG, Gardner MJ. Confidence intervals for research findings. *Br J Obstet Gynecol* 1992;**99**:90–1.
11 Grimes DA. The case for confidence intervals. *Obstet Gynecol* 1992;**80**:865–6.
12 Scialli AR. Confidence and the null hypothesis. *Reprod Toxicol* 1992;**6**:383–4.
13 Harris EK. On P values and confidence intervals (why can't we P with more confidence?) *Clin Chem* 1993;**39**:927–8.
14 Hollis S. Statistics in *Diabetic Medicine*: how confident can you be? *Diabetic Med* 1993;**10**:103–4.
15 Potter RH. Significance level and confidence interval. *J Dent Res* 1994;**73**:494–6.
16 Waller PC, Jackson PR, Tucker GT, Ramsay LE. Clinical pharmacology with confidence. *Br J Clin Pharmacol* 1994;**37**:309–10.
17 Altman DG. Use of confidence intervals to indicate uncertainty in research findings. *Evidence-Based Med* 1996;**1** (May–June): 102–4.
18 Northridge ME, Levin B, Feinleib M, Susser MW. Statistics in the journal – significance, confidence and all that. *Am J Public Health* 1997;**87**:1092–5.
19 Sim J, Reid N. Statistical inference by confidence intervals: issues of interpretation and utilization. *Phys Ther* 1999;**79**:186–95.
20 Kelbæk HS, Gjørup T, Hilden J. Sikkerhedsintervaller i stedet for P-værdier. *Ugeskr Læger* 1990;**152**:2623–8.
21 Chinn S. Statistics in respiratory medicine. 1. Ranges, confidence intervals and related quantities: what they are and when to use them. *Thorax* 1991;**46**:391–3.
22 Borenstein M. A note on the use of confidence intervals in psychiatric research. *Psychopharmacol Bull* 1994;**30**:235–8.
23 Healy MJR. Size, power, and confidence. *Arch Dis Child* 1992;**67**:1495–7.
24 Dorey F, Nasser S, Amstutz H. The need for confidence intervals in the presentation of orthopaedic data. *J Bone Joint Surg* 1993;**75A**:1844–52.
25 Birnbaum D, Sheps SB. The merits of confidence intervals relative to hypothesis testing. *Infect Control Hosp Epidemiol* 1992;**13**:553–5.
25a Henderson AR. Chemistry with confidence: should *Clinical Chemistry* require confidence intervals for analytical and other data? *Clin Chem* 1993;**39**:929–35.
26 Metz CE. Quantification of failure to demonstrate statistical significance. *Invest Radiol* 1993:**28**:59–63.

27 Borenstein M. Hypothesis testing and effect size estimation in clinical trials. *Ann Allergy Asthma Immunol* 1997;**78**:5–11.
28 Young KD, Lewis RJ. What is confidence? Part 1: The use and interpretation of confidence intervals. *Ann Emerg Med* 1997;**30**:307–10.
29 Young KD, Lewis RJ. What is confidence? Part 2: Detailed definition and determination of confidence intervals. *Ann Emerg Med* 1997;**30**:311–18.
30 Greenfield MVH, Kuhn JE, Wojtys EM. A statistics primer. Confidence intervals. *Am J Sports Med* 1998;**26**:145–9.
31 Fitzmaurice G. Confidence intervals. *Nutrition* 1999;**15**:515–16.
32 International Committee of Medical Journal Editors. Uniform Requirements for Manuscripts Submitted to Biomedical Journals. *BMJ* 1988;**296**:401–5.
33 International Committee of Medical Journal Editors. Uniform Requirements for Manuscripts Submitted to Biomedical Journals. *Ann Intern Med* 1997; **126**:36–47 (see also http://www.acponline.org/journals/resource/unifreqr.htm dated May 1999 – accessed 23 September 1999).
34 Bailar JC, Mosteller F. Guidelines for statistical reporting in articles for medical journals. Amplifications and explanations. *Ann Intern Med* 1988; **108**:266–73.
35 Anonymous. Statistical guidelines for *Diabetic Medicine*. *Diabetic Med* 1993;**10**: 93–4.
36 Diabetic Medicine. Instructions for Authors. http://www.blacksci.co.uk/ (accessed 23 September 1999).
37 Rothman KJ. A show of confidence. *N Eng J Med* 1978;**299**:1362–3.
38 Rothman KJ. Significance questing. *Ann Intern Med* 1986;**105**:445–7.
39 Rothman KJ. Writing for *Epidemiology*. *Epidemiology* 1998;**9**. See also http://www.epidem.com.
40 Lang JM, Rothman KJ, Cann CI. The confounded P value. *Epidemiology* 1998;**9**:7–8.
41 Pitkin RM, Branagan MA. Can the accuracy of abstracts be improved by providing specific instructions? A randomized controlled trial. *JAMA* 1998;**280**: 267–9.
42 Haynes RB, Mulrow CD, Huth EJ, Altman DG, Gardner MJ. More informative abstracts revisited. *Ann Intern Med* 1990;**113**:69–76.
43 Begg C, Cho M, Eastwood S, Horton R, Moher D, Olkin I, *et al*. Improving the quality of reporting of randomized controlled trials: the CONSORT statement. *JAMA* 1996;**276**:637–9.
44 Altman DG. Statistical reviewing for medical journals. *Stat Med* 1998;**17**: 2662–74.
45 Deeks JJ, Altman DG. Sensitivity and specificity and their confidence intervals cannot exceed 100%. *BMJ* 1999;**318**:193–4.
46 Altman DG. ROC curves and confidence intervals: getting them right. *Heart* 2000;**83**:236.
47 Hawkins DF. Clinical trials – meta-analysis, confidence limits and 'intention to treat' analysis. *J Obstet Gynaecol* 1990;**10**:259–60.
48 Charlton BG. The future of clinical research: from megatrials towards methodological rigour and representative sampling. *J Eval Clin Practice* 1996; **2**:159–69.
49 Hilden J. Book review of Lang TA, Secic M, 'How to report statistics in medicine. Annotated guidelines for authors, editors and reviewers'. *Med Decis Making* 1998;**18**:351–2.
50 Hall DB. Confidence intervals and controlled clinical trials: incompatible tools for medical research. *J Biopharmaceut Stat* 1993;**3**:257–63.
51 Braitman LE. Statistical estimates and clinical trials. *J Biopharmaceut Stat* 1993;**3**:249–56.
52 Simon R. Why confidence intervals are useful tools in clinical therapeutics. *J Biopharmaceut Stat* 1993;**3**:243–8.

53 Borenstein M. The case for confidence intervals in controlled clinical trials. *Controlled Clin Trials* 1994;**15**:411–28.

54 Altman DG, Bland JM. Absence of evidence is not evidence of absence. *BMJ* 1995;**311**:485.

55 Moher D, Cook DJ, Eastwood S, Olkin I, Rennie D, Stroup DF, *et al.* Improving the quality of reports of meta-analyses of randomized controlled trials: the QUOROM statement. *Lancet*, in press.

56 Freeman PR. The role of P-values in analysing trial results. *Stat Med* 1993;**12**:1443–52.

57 Feinstein AR. P-values and confidence intervals: two sides to the same unsatisfactory coin. *J Clin Epidemiol* 1998;**51**:355–60.

58 Savitz DA. Is statistical significance testing useful in interpreting data? *Reprod Toxicol* 1993;**7**:95–100.

59 Burton PR, Gurrin LC, Campbell MJ. Clinical significance not statistical significance: a simple Bayesian alternative to P values. *J Epidemiol Community Health* 1998;**52**:318–23.

60 Goodman SN. Towards evidence-based medical statistics. Part 1. The P value fallacy. *Ann Intern Med* 1999;**130**:995–1004.

61 Goodman SN. Towards evidence-based medical statistics. Part 2. The Bayes factor. *Ann Intern Med* 1999;**130**:1005–21.

3 Confidence intervals rather than P values

MARTIN J GARDNER, DOUGLAS G ALTMAN

Summary

- Overemphasis on hypothesis testing—and the use of P values to dichotomise results as significant or non-significant—has detracted from more useful approaches to interpreting study results, such as estimation and confidence intervals.
- In medical studies investigators should usually be interested in determining the size of difference of a measured outcome between groups, rather than a simple indication of whether or not it is statistically significant.
- Confidence intervals present a range of values, on the basis of the sample data, in which the population value for such a difference is likely to lie.
- Confidence intervals, if appropriate to the type of study, should be used for major findings in both the main text of a paper and its abstract.

Introduction

Over recent decades the use of statistics in medical journals has increased tremendously. One unfortunate consequence has been a shift in emphasis away from the basic results towards an undue concentration on hypothesis testing. In this approach data are examined in relation to a statistical "null" hypothesis, and the practice has led to the mistaken belief that studies should aim at obtaining "statistical significance". On the contrary, the purpose of most research investigations in medicine is to determine the magnitude of some factor(s) of interest. For example, a laboratory-based study may investigate the difference in mean concentrations of a blood constituent between patients with and without a certain illness, while a clinical study may assess the difference in prognosis of patients with a particular disease treated by alternative regimens in terms of rates of cure, remission, relapse, survival, etc. The difference obtained in such a study will be only an estimate of what we really need, which is the result that would have been obtained had all the eligible subjects (the "population") been investigated rather than just a sample of them. What authors and readers should want to know is by how much the illness modified the mean blood concentrations or by how much the new treatment altered the prognosis, rather than only the level of statistical significance.

The excessive use of hypothesis testing at the expense of other ways of assessing results has reached such a degree that levels of significance are often quoted alone in the main text and abstracts of papers, with no mention of actual concentrations, proportions, etc., or their differences. The implication of hypothesis testing—that there can always be a simple "yes" or "no" answer as the fundamental result from a medical study—is clearly false and used in this way hypothesis testing is of limited value (see chapter 14).

We discuss here the rationale behind an alternative statistical approach—the use of confidence intervals; these are more informative than P values, and we recommend them for papers presenting research findings. This should not be taken to mean that confidence intervals should appear in all papers; in some cases, such as where the data are purely descriptive, confidence intervals are inappropriate and in others techniques for obtaining them are complex or unavailable.

Presentation of study results: limitations of P values

The common simple statements "P < 0·05", "P > 0·05", or "P = NS" convey little information about a study's findings and rely on an arbitrary convention of using the 5% level of statistical significance to define two alternative outcomes—significant or not significant—which is not helpful and encourages lazy thinking. Furthermore, even precise P values convey nothing about the sizes of the differences between study groups. Rothman pointed this out in 1978 and advocated the use of confidence intervals,[1] and in 1984 he and his colleagues repeated the proposal.[2] This plea has been echoed by many others since (see chapter 2).

Presenting P values alone can lead to their being given more merit than they deserve. In particular, there is a tendency to equate statistical significance with medical importance or biological relevance. But small differences of no real interest can be statistically significant with large sample sizes, whereas clinically important effects may be statistically non-significant only because the number of subjects studied was small.

Presentation of study results: confidence intervals

It is more useful to present sample statistics as estimates of results that would be obtained if the total population were studied. The lack of precision of a sample statistic—for example, the mean—which results from both the degree of variability in the factor being investigated and the limited size of the study, can be shown advantageously by a confidence interval.

A confidence interval produces a move from a single value estimate—such as the sample mean, difference between sample means, etc.—to a range of values that are considered to be plausible for the population. The width of a confidence interval associated with a sample statistic depends partly on its standard error, and hence on both the standard deviation and the sample size (see appendix 1 for a brief description of the important, but often misunderstood, distinction between the standard deviation and standard error). It also depends on the degree of "confidence" that we want to associate with the resulting interval.

Suppose that in a study comparing samples of 100 diabetic and 100 non-diabetic men of a certain age a difference of 6·0 mmHg was found between their mean systolic blood pressures and that the standard error of this difference between sample means was 2·5 mmHg, comparable to the difference between means in the Framingham study.[3] The 95% confidence interval for the population difference between means is from 1·1 to 10·9 mmHg and is shown in Figure 3.1 together with the original data. Details of how to calculate the confidence interval are given in chapter 4.

Put simply, this means that there is a 95% chance that the indicated range includes the "population" difference in mean blood pressure levels—that is, the value which would be obtained by including the total populations of diabetics and non-diabetics at which the study is aimed. More exactly, in a statistical sense, the

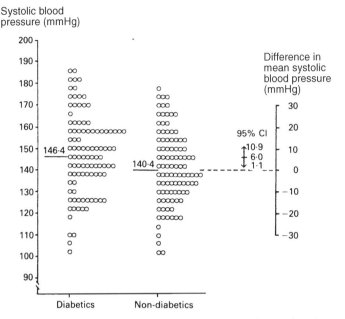

Figure 3.1 Systolic blood pressures in 100 diabetics and 100 non-diabetics with mean levels of 146·4 and 140·4 mmHg respectively. The difference between the sample means of 6.0 mmHg is shown to the right together with the 95% confidence interval from 1·1 to 10·9 mmHg.

confidence interval means that if a series of identical studies were carried out repeatedly on different samples from the same populations, and a 95% confidence interval for the difference between the sample means calculated in each study, then, in the long run, 95% of these confidence intervals would include the population difference between means.

The sample size affects the size of the standard error and this in turn affects the width of the confidence interval. This is shown in Figure 3.2, which shows the 95% confidence interval from samples with the same means and standard deviations as before but only half as large—that is, 50 diabetics and 50 non-diabetics. Reducing the sample size leads to less precision and an increase in the width of the confidence interval, in this case by some 40%.

The investigator can select the degree of confidence associated with a confidence interval, though 95% is the most common choice—just as a 5% level of statistical significance is widely

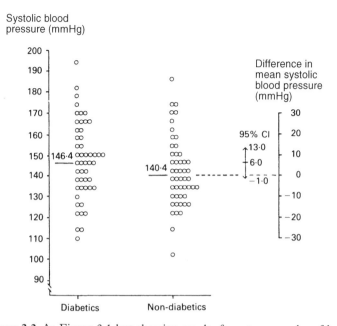

Figure 3.2 As Figure 3.1 but showing results from two samples of half the size—that is, 50 subjects each. The means and standard deviations are as in fig 3.1, but the 95% confidence interval is wider, from −1·0 to 13·0 mmHg, owing to the smaller sample sizes.

used. If greater or less confidence is required different intervals can be constructed: 99%, 95%, and 90% confidence intervals for the data in Figure 3.1 are shown in Figure 3.3. As would be expected, greater confidence that the population difference is within a confidence interval is obtained with wider intervals. In practice, intervals other than 99%, 95%, or 90% are rarely quoted. Appendix 2 explains the general method for calculating a confidence interval appropriate for most of the methods described in this book. In brief, a confidence interval is obtained by subtracting from, and adding to, the estimated statistic of interest (such as a mean difference) a multiple of its standard error (SE). A few methods described in this book, however, do not follow this pattern.

Confidence intervals convey only the effects of sampling variation on the precision of the estimated statistics and cannot control for non-sampling errors such as biases in design, conduct, or analysis.

19

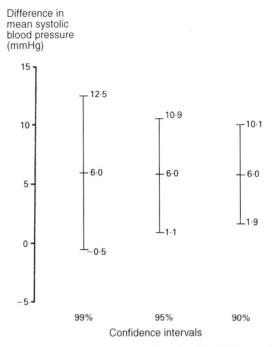

Figure 3.3 Confidence intervals associated with differing degrees of "confidence" using the same data as in Figure 3.1.

Sample sizes and confidence intervals

In general, increasing the sample size will reduce the width of the confidence interval. If we assume the same means and standard deviations as in the example, Figure 3.4 shows the resulting 99%, 95%, and 90% confidence intervals for the difference in mean blood pressures for sample sizes of up to 500 in each group. The benefit, in terms of narrowing the confidence interval, of a further increase in the number of subjects, falls sharply with increasing sample size. Similar effects occur in estimating other statistics such as proportions.

For a total study sample size of N subjects, the confidence interval for the difference in population means is narrowest when both groups are of size $N/2$. However, the width of the confidence interval will be only slightly larger with differing numbers in each group unless one group size is relatively small.

During the planning stage of a study it is possible to estimate the sample size that should be used by stating the width of the

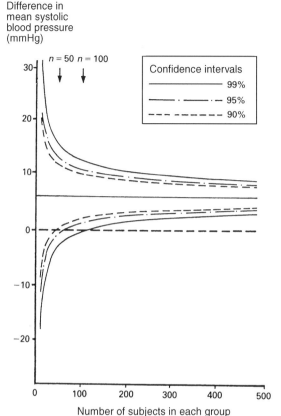

Figure 3.4 Confidence intervals resulting from the same means and standard deviations as in Figure 3.1 but showing the effect on the confidence interval of sample sizes of up to 500 subjects in each group. The two horizontal lines show: - - - - zero difference between means, —— observed study difference between means of 6·0 mmHg. The arrows indicate the confidence intervals shown in Figures 3.1–3.3 for sample sizes of 100 and 50 in each group.

confidence interval required at the end of the study and carrying out the appropriate calculation (see chapter 12).

Confidence intervals and statistical significance

There is a close link between the use of a confidence interval and a two-sided hypothesis test. If the confidence interval is calculated then the result of the hypothesis test (often less accurately referred to as a significance test) can be inferred at an associated level of statistical significance. The right-hand scale in Figure 3.1 includes the point that represents a zero difference in mean blood pressure between diabetics and non-diabetics. This zero difference between means corresponds to the value examined under the "null hypothesis" and, as Figure 3.1 shows, it is outside the 95% confidence interval. This indicates that a statistically significant difference between the sample means at the 5% level would result from applying the appropriate unpaired t test. Figure 3.3, however, shows that the P value is greater than 1% because zero is inside the 99% confidence interval, so $0.01 < P < 0.05$. By contrast, had zero been within the 95% confidence interval this would have indicated a non-significant result at the 5% level. Such an example is shown in Figure 3.2 for the smaller samples.

The 95% confidence interval covers a wide range of possible population mean differences, even though the sample difference between means is different from zero at the 5% level of statistical significance. In particular, the 95% confidence interval shows that the study result is compatible with a small difference of around 1 mmHg as well as with a difference as great as 10 mmHg in mean blood pressures. Nevertheless, the difference between population means is much more likely to be near to the middle of the confidence interval than towards the extremes. Although the confidence interval is wide, the best estimate of the population difference is 6·0 mmHg, the difference between the sample means.

This example therefore shows the lack of precision of the observed sample difference between means as an estimate of the population value, and this is clear in each of the three confidence intervals shown in Figure 3.3. It also shows the weakness of considering statistical significance in isolation from the numerical estimates.

The confidence interval thus provides a range of possibilities for the population value, rather than an arbitrary dichotomy based solely on statistical significance. It conveys more useful information at the expense of precision of the P value. However, the actual P value is helpful in addition to the confidence interval, and preferably both should be presented. If one has to be excluded, however, it should be the P value.

Suggested mode of presentation

In content, our only proposed change is that confidence intervals should be reported instead of standard errors. This will encourage a move away from the emphasis on statistical significance. For the major finding(s) of a study we recommend that full statistical information should be given, including sample estimates, confidence intervals, test statistics, and P values—assuming that basic details, such as sample sizes and standard deviations, have been reported earlier in the paper. The major findings would include at least those related to the original hypothesis(es) of the study and those reported in the abstract.

For the above example the textual presentation of the results might read:

> The difference between the sample mean systolic blood pressures in diabetics and non-diabetics was 6·0 mmHg, with a 95% confidence interval from 1·1 to 10·9 mmHg; the t test statistic was 2·4, with 198 degrees of freedom and an associated P value of 0·02.

In short:

> Mean 6·0 mmHg, 95% confidence interval 1·1 to 10·9; $t = 2·4$, df = 198, P = 0·02.

It is preferable to use the word "to" for separating the two values rather than a dash, as a dash is confusing when at least one of the numbers is negative. The use of the $\pm$ sign should also be avoided (see appendix 1 and chapter 14). The exact P value from the t distribution is 0·01732, but one or two significant figures are enough (see chapter 14); this value is seen to be within the range 0·01 to 0·05 determined earlier from the confidence intervals.

The two extremes of a confidence interval are known as confidence limits. However, the word "limits" suggests that there is no going beyond and may be misunderstood because, of course, the population value will not always lie within the confidence interval. Moreover, there is a danger that one or other of the "limits" will be quoted in isolation from the rest of the results, with misleading consequences. For example, concentrating only on the larger limit and ignoring the rest of the confidence interval would misrepresent the finding by exaggerating the study difference. Conversely, quoting only the smaller limit would incorrectly underestimate the difference. The confidence interval is thus preferable because it focuses on the range of values.

The same notation can be used for presenting confidence intervals in tables. Thus, a column headed "95% confidence interval" or "95% CI" would have rows of intervals: 1·1 to 10·9, 48 to 85, etc. Confidence intervals can also be incorporated into figures, where they are preferable to the widely used standard error, which is often shown solely in one direction from the sample estimate. If individual data values can be shown as well, which is usually possible for small samples, this is even more informative. Thus in Figure 3.1, despite the considerable overlap of the two sets of sample data, the shift in means is shown by the 95% confidence interval excluding zero. For paired samples, the individual differences can be plotted advantageously in a diagram.

The example given here of the difference between two means is common. Although there is some intrinsic interest in the mean values themselves, inferences from a study will be concerned mainly with their difference. Giving confidence intervals for each mean separately is therefore unhelpful, because these do not indicate the precision of the difference or its statistical significance.[4,5] Thus, the major contrasts of a study should be shown directly, rather than only vaguely in terms of the separate means (or proportions).

For a paper with only a limited number of statistical comparisons related to the initial hypotheses, confidence intervals are recommended throughout. Where multiple comparisons are concerned, however, the usual problems of interpretation arise, since some confidence intervals will exclude the "null" value—for example, zero difference—through random sampling variation alone. This mirrors the situation of calculating a multiplicity of P values, where not all statistically significant differences are likely to represent real effects[6] (see chapter 13). Judgement needs to be exercised over the number of statistical comparisons made, with confidence intervals and P values calculated, to avoid misleading both authors and readers (see chapter 14).

Conclusion

The excessive use of hypothesis testing at the expense of more informative approaches to data interpretation is an unsatisfactory way of assessing and presenting statistical findings from medical studies. We prefer the use of confidence intervals, which present the results directly on the scale of data measurement. We have also suggested a notation for confidence intervals which is intended to force clarity of meaning.

Confidence intervals, which also have a link to the outcome of hypothesis tests, should become the standard method for presenting the statistical results of major findings.

Appendix 1: Standard deviation and standard error

When numerical findings are reported, regardless of whether or not their statistical significance is quoted, they are often presented with additional statistical information. The distinction between two widely quoted statistics—the standard deviation and the standard error—is, however, often misunderstood.[7-12]

The standard deviation is a measure of the variability between individuals in the level of the factor being investigated, such as blood alcohol concentrations in a sample of car drivers, and is thus a descriptive index. By contrast, the standard error is a measure of the uncertainty in a sample statistic. For example, the standard error of the mean indicates the uncertainty of the mean blood alcohol concentration among the sample of drivers as an estimate of the mean value among the population of all car drivers. The standard deviation is relevant when variability between individuals is of interest; the standard error is relevant to summary statistics such as means, proportions, differences, regression slopes, etc. (see chapter 14).

The standard error of the sample statistic, which depends on both the standard deviation and the sample size, is a recognition that a sample is most unlikely to determine the population value exactly. In fact, if a further sample is taken in identical circumstances almost certainly it will produce a different estimate of the same population value. The sample statistic is therefore imprecise, and the standard error is a measure of this imprecision. By itself the standard error has limited meaning, but it can be used to produce a confidence interval, which does have a useful interpretation.

In many publications a $\pm$ sign is used to join the standard deviation (SD) or standard error (SE) to an observed mean—for example, $69 \cdot 4 \pm 9 \cdot 3$ kg—but the notation gives no indication whether the second figure is the standard deviation or the standard error (or something else).[12] As is suggested in chapter 14, a clearer presentation would be in the unambiguous form "the mean was $69 \cdot 4$ kg (SD $9 \cdot 3$ kg)". The present policy of the *BMJ* and many other journals is to remove $\pm$ signs and request authors to indicate clearly whether the standard deviation or standard error is being quoted. All journals should follow this practice;[13] it avoids any possible misunderstanding from the omission of SD or SE.[14]

Appendix 2: Constructing confidence intervals

Frequently we can reasonably assume that the estimate of interest, such as the difference between two proportions (see chapter 6), has a Normal sampling distribution. To construct a confidence interval for the population value we are interested in the range of values within which the sample estimate would fall on most occasions (see main text of this chapter). The calculation of confidence intervals is simplified by the ability to convert the standard Normal distribution into the Normal distribution of interest by multiplying by the standard error of the estimate and adding the value of the estimate.

To construct a 95% confidence interval, say, we use the central 95% of the standard Normal distribution, so we need the values that cut off 2·5% of the distribution at each end (or "tail"). Thus we need the values of $z_{0.025}$ and $z_{0.975}$. In general we construct a $100(1 - \alpha)\%$ confidence interval using the values $z_{\alpha/2}$ and $z_{1-\alpha/2}$ which cut off the bottom and top $100\alpha/2\%$ of the distribution. Figure 3.5 illustrates the procedure.

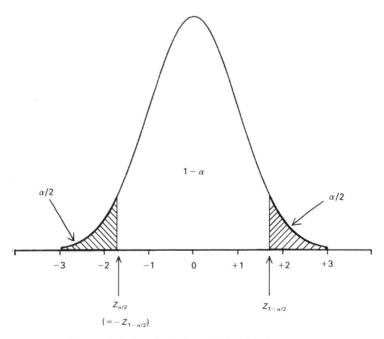

Figure 3.5 Standard Normal distribution curve.

To convert back to the scale of the original data we multiply the two values $z_{\alpha/2}$ and $z_{1-\alpha/2}$ by the standard error (SE) and add them to the estimate, to get the $100(1-\alpha)\%$ confidence interval as

$$\text{estimate} + (z_{\alpha/2} \times \text{SE}) \quad \text{to} \quad \text{estimate} + (z_{1-\alpha/2} \times \text{SE}).$$

As explained in the notation list at the end of the book (chapter 16), an equivalent expression is

$$\text{estimate} - (z_{1-\alpha/2} \times \text{SE}) \quad \text{to} \quad \text{estimate} + (z_{1-\alpha/2} \times \text{SE})$$

which makes explicit the symmetry of the confidence interval around the estimate.

For some estimates, such as the difference between sample means (see chapter 4), the appropriate sampling distribution is the t distribution. Exactly the same procedure is adopted but with $z_{1-\alpha/2}$ replaced by $t_{1-\alpha/2}$. For other estimates different sampling distributions are relevant, such as the Poisson distribution for standardised mortality ratios (see chapter 7) or the Binomial for medians (see chapter 5).

1 Rothman KJ. A show of confidence. *N Engl J Med* 1978;**299**:1362–3.
2 Poole C, Lanes S, Rothman KJ. Analysing data from ordered categories. *N Engl J Med* 1984;**311**:1382.
3 Kannel WB, McGee DL. Diabetes and cardiovascular risk factors: the Framingham study. *Circulation* 1979;**59**:8–13.
4 Browne RH. On visual assessment of the significance of a mean difference. *Biometrics* 1979;**35**:657–65.
5 Altman DG. Statistics and ethics in medical research: VI—presentation of results. *BMJ* 1980;**281**:1542–4.
6 Jones, DR, Rushton L. Simultaneous inference in epidemiological studies. *Int J Epidemiol* 1982;**11**:276–82.
7 Gardner MJ. Understanding and presenting variation. *Lancet* 1975;**i**:230–1.
8 Feinstein AR. Clinical biostatistics XXXVII: demeaned errors, confidence games, nonplussed minuses, inefficient coefficients, and other statistical disruptions of scientific communication. *Clin Pharmacol Ther* 1976;**20**:617–31.
9 Bunce H, Hokanson JA, Weiss GB. Avoiding ambiguity when reporting variability in biomedical data. *Am J Med* 1980;**69**:8–9.
10 Altman DG. Statistics in medical journals. *Stat Med* 1982;**1**:59–71.
11 Brown GW. Standard deviation, standard error: which "standard"should we use? *Am J Dis Child* 1982;**136**:937–41.
12 Altman DG, Gardner MJ. Presentation of variability. *Lancet* 1986;**ii**:639.
13 Huth EJ. Uniform requirements for manuscripts: the new, third edition. *Ann Intern Med* 1988;**108**:298–9.
14 Bailar JC, Mosteller F. Guidelines for statistical reporting in articles for medical journals: amplifications and explanations. *Ann Intern Med* 1988;**108**:266–73.

4 Means and their differences

DOUGLAS G ALTMAN, MARTIN J GARDNER

The rationale behind the use of confidence intervals was described in chapters 1 and 3. Here formulae for calculating confidence intervals are given for means and their differences. There is a common underlying principle of subtracting and adding to the sample statistic a multiple of its standard error (SE). This extends to other statistics, such as proportions and regression coefficients, but is not universal.

Confidence intervals for means are constructed using the t distribution if the data have an approximately Normal distribution. For differences between two means the data should also have similar standard deviations (SDs) in each study group. This is implicit in the example given in chapter 3 and in the worked examples below. The calculations have been carried out to full arithmetical precision, as is recommended practice (see chapter 14), but intermediate steps are shown as rounded results.

The case of non-Normal data is discussed both in this chapter and in chapter 5.

A confidence interval indicates the precision of the sample mean or the difference between two sample means as an estimate of the overall population value. As such, confidence intervals convey the effects of sampling variation but cannot control for nonsampling errors in study design or conduct.

Single sample

The confidence interval for a population mean is derived using the mean $\bar{x}$ and its standard error $SE(\bar{x})$ from a sample of size n. For this case the standard error is obtained simply from the sample standard deviation (SD) as $SE = SD/\sqrt{n}$. Thus, the confidence interval is given by

$$\bar{x} - [t_{1-\alpha/2} \times \mathrm{SE}(\bar{x})] \quad \text{to} \quad \bar{x} + [t_{1-\alpha/2} \times \mathrm{SE}(\bar{x})]$$

where $t_{1-\alpha/2}$ is the appropriate value from the t distribution with $n-1$ degrees of freedom associated with a "confidence" of $100(1-\alpha)\%$. For a 95% confidence interval α is 0.05, for a 99% confidence interval α is 0.01, and so on. Values of t can be found from Table 18.2 or in statistical textbooks.[1,2] For a 95% confidence interval the value of t will be close to 2 for samples of 20 upwards but noticeably greater than 2 for smaller samples.

Worked example

Blood pressure levels were measured in a sample of 100 diabetic men aged 40–49 years. The mean systolic blood pressure was $146.4\,\mathrm{mmHg}$ and the standard deviation $18.5\,\mathrm{mmHg}$. The standard error of the mean is thus found as $18.5/\sqrt{100} = 1.85$.

To calculate the 95% confidence interval the appropriate value of $t_{0.975}$ with 99 degrees of freedom is 1.984. The 95% confidence interval for the population value of the mean systolic blood pressure is then given by

$$146.4 - (1.984 \times 1.85) \quad \text{to} \quad 146.4 + (1.984 \times 1.85)$$

that is, from 142.7 to $150.1\,\mathrm{mmHg}$.

Two samples: unpaired case

The confidence interval for the difference between two population means is derived in a similar way. Suppose $\bar{x}_1$ and $\bar{x}_2$ are the two sample means, s_1 and s_2 the corresponding standard deviations, and n_1 and n_2 the sample sizes. Firstly, we need a "pooled" estimate of the standard deviation, which is given by

$$s = \sqrt{\frac{(n_1 - 1)s_1^2 + (n_2 - 1)s_2^2}{n_1 + n_2 - 2}}.$$

From this the standard error of the difference between the two sample means is

$$\mathrm{SE}(d) = s \times \sqrt{\frac{1}{n_1} + \frac{1}{n_2}}$$

where $d = \bar{x}_1 - \bar{x}_2$. The $100(1-\alpha)\%$ confidence interval for the difference in the two population means is then

$$d - [t_{1-\alpha/2} \times \mathrm{SE}(d)] \quad \text{to} \quad d + [t_{1-\alpha/2} \times \mathrm{SE}(d)],$$

where $t_{1-\alpha/2}$ is taken from the t distribution with $n_1 + n_2 - 2$ degrees of freedom (see Table 18.2).

If the standard deviations differ considerably then a common pooled estimate is not appropriate unless a suitable transformation of scale can be found.[3] Otherwise obtaining a confidence interval is more complex.[4]

Worked example

Blood pressure levels were measured in 100 diabetic and 100 non-diabetic men aged 40–49 years. Mean systolic blood pressures were 146·4 mmHg (SD 18·5) among the diabetics and 140·4 mmHg (SD 16·8) among the non-diabetics, giving a difference between sample means of 6·0 mmHg.

Using the formulae given above the pooled estimate of the standard deviation is

$$s = \sqrt{\frac{(99 \times 18 \cdot 5^2) + (99 \times 16 \cdot 8^2)}{198}} = 17 \cdot 7 \, \text{mmHg}$$

and the standard error of the difference between the sample means is

$$\text{SE}(d) = 17 \cdot 7 \times \sqrt{\frac{1}{100} + \frac{1}{100}} = 2 \cdot 50 \, \text{mmHg}.$$

To calculate the 95% confidence interval the appropriate value of $t_{1-\alpha/2}$ with 198 degrees of freedom is 1·972. Thus the 95% confidence interval for the difference in population means is given by

$$6 \cdot 0 - (1 \cdot 972 \times 2 \cdot 50) \quad \text{to} \quad 6 \cdot 0 + (1 \cdot 972 \times 2 \cdot 50)$$

that is, from 1·1 to 10·9 mmHg, as shown in Figure 3.1.

Suppose now that the samples had been of only 50 men each but that the means and standard deviations had been the same. Then the pooled standard deviation would remain 17·7 mmHg, but the standard error of the difference between the sample means would become

$$\text{SE}(d) = 17 \cdot 7 \times \sqrt{\frac{1}{50} + \frac{1}{50}} = 3 \cdot 53 \, \text{mmHg}.$$

The appropriate value of $t_{1-\alpha/2}$ on 98 degrees of freedom is 1·984, and the 95% confidence interval is calculated as

$$6 \cdot 0 - (1 \cdot 984 \times 3 \cdot 53) \quad \text{to} \quad 6 \cdot 0 + (1 \cdot 984 \times 3 \cdot 53)$$

that is, from −1·0 to 13·0 mmHg, as shown in Figure 3.2.

For the original samples of 100 each the appropriate values of $t_{0.995}$ and $t_{0.95}$ with 198 degrees of freedom to calculate the 99% and 90% confidence intervals are 2·601 and 1·653, respectively. Thus the 99% confidence interval is calculated as

$$6 \cdot 0 - (2 \cdot 601 \times 2 \cdot 50) \quad \text{to} \quad 6 \cdot 0 + (2 \cdot 601 \times 2 \cdot 50)$$

that is, from -0.5 to 12.5 mmHg (Figure 3.3), and the 90% confidence interval is given by

$$6.0 - (1.653 \times 2.50) \quad \text{to} \quad 6.0 + (1.653 \times 2.50)$$

that is, from 1.9 to 10.1 mmHg (Figure 3.3).

Two samples: paired case

Paired data arise in studies of repeated measurements—for example, at different times or in different circumstances on the same subjects—and matched case-control comparisons. For such data the same formulae as for the single sample case are used to calculate the confidence interval, where $\bar{x}$ and SD are now the mean and standard deviation of the individual within subject or patient–control differences.

Worked example

Systolic blood pressure levels were measured in 16 middle-aged men before and after a standard exercise, giving the results shown in Table 4.1.

The mean difference (rise) in systolic blood pressure following exercise was 6.6 mmHg. The standard deviation of the differences, shown in the last column of Table 4.1, is 6.0 mmHg. Thus the standard error of the mean difference is found as $6.0/\sqrt{16} = 1.49$ mmHg.

Table 4.1 Systolic blood pressure levels (mmHg) in 16 men before and after exercise

Subject number	Systolic blood pressure (mmHg)		Difference After − before
	Before	After	
1	148	152	+4
2	142	152	+10
3	136	134	−2
4	134	148	+14
5	138	144	+6
6	140	136	−4
7	132	144	+12
8	144	150	+6
9	128	146	+18
10	170	174	+4
11	162	162	0
12	150	162	+12
13	138	146	+8
14	154	156	+2
15	126	132	+6
16	116	126	+10

To calculate the 95% confidence interval the appropriate value of $t_{0.975}$ with 15 degrees of freedom is 2·131. The 95% confidence interval for the population value of the mean systolic blood pressure increase after the standard exercise is then given by

$$6·6 - (2·131 \times 1·49) \quad \text{to} \quad 6·6 + (2·131 \times 1·49)$$

that is, from 3·4 to 9·8 mmHg.

Non-Normal data

The sample data may have to be transformed on to a different scale to achieve approximate Normality. The most common reason is because the distribution of the observations is skewed, with a long "tail" of high values. The logarithmic transformation is the most frequently used. Transformation often also helps to make the standard deviations on the transformed scale in different groups more similar.[5]

Single sample

For a single sample a mean and confidence interval can be constructed from the transformed data and then transformed back to the original scale of measurement.[6] This is preferable to presenting the results in units of, say, log mmHg. With highly skewed or otherwise awkward data the median may be preferable to the mean as a measure of central tendency and used with non-parametric methods of analysis. Confidence intervals can be calculated for the median (see chapter 5).

Worked example

Table 4.2 shows T4 and T8 lymphocyte counts in 28 haemophiliacs[7] ranked in increasing order of the T4 counts.

Suppose that we wish to calculate a confidence interval for the mean T4 lymphocyte count in the population of haemophiliacs. Inspection of histograms and plots of the data reveals that whereas the distribution of T4 values is skewed, after logarithmic transformation the values of $\log_e$ (T4) have a symmetric near Normal distribution. We can thus apply the method given previously for calculating a confidence interval for a population mean derived from a single sample of observations.

The mean of the values of $\log_e$ (T4) is −0·2896 and the standard deviation is 0·5921. Thus the standard error of the mean is found as $0·5921/\sqrt{28} = 0·1119$. The units here are log lymphocyte counts × 10^9/l.

To calculate the 95% confidence interval the appropriate value of $t_{0.975}$ with 27 degrees of freedom is 2·052. The 95% confidence interval for the

Table 4.2 T4 and T8 lymphocyte counts ($\times 10^9$/l) in 28 haemophiliacs[7]

Subject number	T4	T8	$\log_e$ (T4) $-$ $\log_e$ (T8)
1	0·20	0·17	0·163
2	0·27	0·52	−0·655
3	0·28	0·25	0·113
4	0·37	0·34	0·085
5	0·38	0·14	0·999
6	0·48	0·10	1·569
7	0·49	0·58	−0·169
8	0·56	0·23	0·890
9	0·60	0·24	0·916
10	0·64	0·67	−0·046
11	0·64	0·90	−0·341
12	0·66	0·26	0·932
13	0·70	0·51	0·317
14	0·77	0·18	1·453
15	0·88	0·74	0·173
16	0·88	0·54	0·488
17	0·88	0·76	0·147
18	0·90	0·62	0·373
19	1·02	0·48	0·754
20	1·10	0·58	0·640
21	1·10	0·34	1·174
22	1·18	0·84	0·340
23	1·20	0·63	0·644
24	1·30	0·46	1·039
25	1·40	0·84	0·511
26	1·60	1·20	0·288
27	1·64	0·59	1·022
28	2·40	1·30	0·613

mean $\log_e$ (T4) in the population is then given by

$$-0{\cdot}2896 - (2{\cdot}052 \times 0{\cdot}1119) \quad \text{to} \quad -0{\cdot}2896 + (2{\cdot}052 \times 0{\cdot}1119)$$

that is, from −0·5192 to −0·0600.

We can transform this confidence interval on the logarithmic scale back to the original units to get a more meaningful confidence interval. First we transform back the mean of $\log_e$ (T4) to get the geometric mean T4 count. This is given as $\exp(-0{\cdot}2896) = 0{\cdot}75 \times 10^9$/l. (The geometric mean is found as the antilog of the mean of the log values.) In the same way we can transform back the values describing the confidence interval to get a 95% confidence interval for the geometric mean T4 lymphocyte count in the population of haemophiliacs, which is thus given by

$$\exp(-0{\cdot}5192) \quad \text{to} \quad \exp(-0{\cdot}0600)$$

that is, from 0·59 to 0·94 $\times 10^9$/l.

Two samples

For the case of two samples, only the logarithmic transformation is suitable.[5] For paired or unpaired samples the confidence interval for the difference in the means of the transformed data has to be transformed back. For the log transformation the antilog of the difference in sample means on the transformed scale is an estimate of the ratio of the two population (geometric) means, and the antilogged confidence interval for the difference gives a confidence interval for this ratio. Other transformations do not lead to sensible confidence intervals when transformed back,[5] but a non-parametric approach can be used to calculate a confidence interval for the population difference between medians (see chapter 5).

Worked example

Suppose that we wish to calculate a confidence interval for the difference between the T4 and T8 counts in the population of haemophiliacs using the results given in Table 4.2. Inspection of histograms and plots of these data reveals that the distribution of the differences T4 − T8 is skewed, but after logarithmic transformation the differences $\log_e (T4) - \log_e (T8)$ have a symmetric near Normal distribution. We can thus apply the method given previously for calculating a confidence interval from paired samples. The method makes use of the fact that the difference between the logarithms of two quantities is exactly the same as the logarithm of their ratio. Thus

$$\log_e (T4) - \log_e (T8) = \log_e (T4/T8).$$

The mean of the differences between the logs of the T4 and T8 counts (shown in the final column of Table 4.2) is 0·5154 and the standard deviation is 0·5276. Thus the standard error of the mean is found as $0·5276/\sqrt{28} = 0·0997$.

To calculate the 95% confidence interval the appropriate value of $t_{0.975}$ with 27 degrees of freedom is 2·052. The 95% confidence interval for the difference between the mean values of $\log_e (T4)$ and $\log_e (T8)$ in the population of haemophiliacs is then given by

$$0·5154 - (2·052 \times 0·0997) \quad \text{to} \quad 0·5154 + (2·052 \times 0·0997)$$

that is, from 0·3108 to 0·7200.

The confidence interval for the difference between log counts is not as easy to interpret as a confidence interval relating to the actual counts. We can take antilogs of the above values to get a more useful confidence interval. The antilog of the mean difference between log counts is $\exp(0·5154) = 1·67$. Because of the equivalence of the difference $\log_e (T4) - \log_e (T8)$ and $\log_e (T4/T8)$ this value is an estimate of the geometric mean of the ratio T4/T8 in the population. The antilogs of the values describing the confidence interval are $\exp(0{\cdot}3108) = 1{\cdot}36$ and $\exp(0{\cdot}7200) = 2{\cdot}05$, and these values provide a 95% confidence interval for the geometric mean ratio of T4 to T8 lymphocyte counts in the population of haemophiliacs.

Note that whereas for a single sample the use of the log transformation still leads to a confidence interval in the original units, for paired samples the confidence interval is in terms of a ratio and has no units.

If log transformation is considered necessary, a confidence interval for the difference in the means of two unpaired samples is derived in much the same way as for paired samples. The log data are used to calculate a confidence interval, using the method for unpaired samples given previously. The antilogs of the difference in the means of the log data and the values describing its confidence interval give the geometric mean ratio and its associated confidence interval.

Comment

The sampling distribution of a mean (and the difference between two means) will become more like a Normal distribution as the sample size increases. However, study sizes typical in medical research are usually not large enough to rely on this property, especially for a single mean, so it is useful to use the log transformation for skewed data. An exception is where one is interested only in the difference between means, not their ratio, such as in studies of cost data.[8]

1 Altman DG. *Practical statistics for medical research*. London: Chapman & Hall, 1991.
2 Campbell MJ, Machin D. *Medical statistics. A commonsense approach*. 3rd edn. Chichester: John Wiley, 1999.
3 Bland JM, Altman DG. Transforming data. *BMJ* 1996;**312**:770.
4 Armitage P, Berry G. *Statistical methods in medical research*. 3rd edn. Oxford: Blackwell Science, 1994:111–14.
5 Bland JM, Altman DG. The use of transformation when comparing two means. *BMJ* 1996;**312**:1153.
6 Bland JM, Altman DG. Transformations, means, and confidence intervals. *BMJ* 1996; **312**:1079.
7 Ball SE, Hows JM, Worslet AM, *et al.* Seroconversion of human T cell lymphotropic virus III (HTLV-III) in patients with haemophilia: a longitudinal study. *BMJ* 1985;**290**:1705–6.
8 Barber JA, Thompson SG. Analysis and interpretation of cost data in randomised controlled trials: review of published studies. *BMJ* 1998;**317**:1195–200.

5 Medians and their differences

MICHAEL J CAMPBELL, MARTIN J GARDNER

The methods for the calculation of confidence intervals for a population mean and for differences between two population means for paired and unpaired samples were given in chapter 4. These methods are based on sample means, standard errors, and the *t* distribution and should strictly be used only for continuous data from Normal distributions (although small deviations from Normality are not important[1]). This is a so-called parametric approach as it essentially estimates the two parameters of the Normal distribution, that is, the mean and standard deviation.

For non-Normal continuous data the median of the population or the sample is often preferable to the mean as a measure of location. This chapter describes methods of calculating confidence intervals for a population median (the 50% quantile) or for other population quantiles from a sample of observations. Calculations of confidence intervals for the difference between two population medians (a non-parametric approach rather than the parametric approach mentioned above) for both unpaired and paired samples are described.

It is a common misapprehension that non-parametric methods are to be preferred if the sample size is small, since distributional assumption cannot be checked in these circumstances. However, non-parametric methods involve a loss of statistical power if Normality assumptions do hold, and so if the sample size is small and if there is good external evidence that the distributions are likely to be of the Normal form, the parametric methods may be preferred.

Because of the discrete nature of some of the sampling distributions involved in non-parametric analyses it is not usually possible to calculate confidence intervals with exactly the desired level of confidence. Hence, if a 95% confidence interval is wanted the choice is between the lowest possible level of confidence over 95% (a "conservative" interval) and the highest possible under 95%. There is no firm policy on which of these is preferred, but we shall mainly describe conservative intervals in this chapter. The exact level of confidence associated with any particular approximate level can be calculated from the distribution of the statistic being used although this may not be very straightforward. Further aspects of conservative and exact confidence intervals are given in chapter 13.

The methods outlined for obtaining confidence intervals are described in more detail in some textbooks on non-parametric statistics (for example, by Conover[2]). If there are many "ties" in the data, that is, observations with the same numerical value, then modifications to the formulae given here are needed.[2] The calculations can be carried out using some statistical computer packages such as MINITAB.[3]

A confidence interval indicates the precision of the sample statistic as an estimate of the overall population value. Confidence intervals convey the effects of sampling variation but cannot control for non-sampling errors in study design or conduct. They should not be used for basic description of the sample data but only for indicating the uncertainty in sample estimates for population values of medians or other statistics.

Medians and other quantiles

Median

The median, M, is defined as the value having half of the observations less than and half exceeding it. It is identified after first ranking the n sample observations in increasing order of magnitude. The sample median is used as an estimate of the population median. To find the $100(1 - \alpha)\%$ confidence interval for the population median first calculate the quantities

$$r = \frac{n}{2} - \left(z_{1-\alpha/2} \times \frac{\sqrt{n}}{2} \right) \quad \text{and} \quad s = 1 + \frac{n}{2} + \left(z_{1-\alpha/2} \times \frac{\sqrt{n}}{2} \right),$$

where $z_{1-\alpha/2}$ is the appropriate value from the standard Normal distribution for the $100(1 - \alpha/2)$ percentile found in Table 18.1. Then round r and s to the nearest integers. The rth and sth observations in the ranking are the $100(1 - \alpha)\%$ confidence interval for the population median.

Worked example

For the data in the first example given in chapter 4 the median systolic blood pressure among 100 diabetic patients was $M = 146\,\text{mmHg}$. Using the above formulae to calculate a 95% confidence interval gives

$$r = \frac{100}{2} - \left(1.96 \times \frac{\sqrt{100}}{2}\right) = 40.2 \quad \text{to}$$

$$s = 1 + \frac{100}{2} + \left(1.96 \times \frac{\sqrt{100}}{2}\right) = 60.8.$$

From the original data the 40th observation in increasing order is 142 mmHg and the 61st is 150 mmHg. The 95% confidence interval for the population median is thus from 142 to 150 mmHg.

This approximate method is satisfactory for most sample sizes.[4] The exact method, based on the Binomial distribution, can be used instead for small samples, as shown in the example below, which uses Table 18.4.

Worked example

The results of a study measuring β-endorphin concentrations in pmol/l in $n = 11$ subjects who had collapsed while running in a half marathon[5] were (in order of increasing value):

66·0, 71·2, 83·0, 83·6, 101·0, 107·6, 122·0, 143·0, 160·0, 177·0, and 414·0.

The sample median is the 6th observation in this ranking, that is $M = 107\cdot6\,\text{pmol/l}$. To find a confidence interval for the population median we use the Binomial distribution[1] with $n = 11$ and probability $\pi = 0\cdot5$. For a conservative 95% confidence interval we first find the largest X, which can take the values $0, 1, 2, \ldots, 11$ which gives the closest cumulative probability under $0\cdot025$ and the smallest X which gives the closest cumulative probability over $0\cdot975$. This can be done either by direct calculation or from tables.[2] This gives Prob $(X \leq 1) = 0\cdot006$ and Prob $(X \leq 9) = 0\cdot994$.

The approximate 95% confidence interval is then found by the ranked observations that are one greater than those associated with the two probabilities, that is, the 2nd and 10th observations, giving 71·2 to 177·0 pmol/l.

The actual probability associated with this confidence interval is in fact $0\cdot994 - 0\cdot006 = 0\cdot988$ rather than $0\cdot95$, so effectively it is a 98·8% confidence interval. For sample sizes up to 100, the required rankings for approximate 90%, 95%, and 99% confidence intervals and associated exact levels of confidence are given directly in Table 18.4.

Alternatively, a non-conservative approximate 95% confidence interval can be found by calculating the smallest cumulative probability over 0·025 and the largest under 0·975. In this case we find Prob $(X \leq 2) = 0\cdot033$ and Prob $(X \leq 8) = 0\cdot967$, which give a $0\cdot967 - 0\cdot033 = 0\cdot935$ or 93·5% confidence interval from the 3rd to the 9th ranked observations, that is, from 83·0 to 160·0 pmol/l.

In this case the coverage probability of 93·5% is nearer to 95% than for the conservative interval coverage of 98·8%.

For this example the approximate large sample method gives a similar result as the conservative 95% confidence interval.

As another alternative, if the population distribution from which the observations came can be assumed to be symmetrical (but not of the Normal distribution shape) rather than skewed around the median, then the method described below in the section "Two samples: paired case" can be used, replacing the differences d_i given there by the sample observations.

Other quantiles

A similar approach can be used to calculate confidence intervals for quantiles other than the median—for example, the 90th percentile, which divides the lower nine tenths from the upper tenth of the observations. For the qth quantile ($q = 0\cdot9$ for the 90th percentile) r and s above are replaced by r_q and s_q given by

$$r_q = nq - [z_{1-\alpha/2} \times \sqrt{nq(1-q)}]$$

and

$$s_q = 1 + nq + [z_{1-\alpha/2} \times \sqrt{nq(1-q)}].$$

Differences between medians

In finding confidence intervals for population differences between medians it is assumed that the data come from distributions that are identical in shape and differ only in location. Because of this assumption the non-parametric confidence intervals described below can be regarded as being either for the difference between the two medians, or the difference between the two means, or the difference between any other two measures of location such as a particular percentile. This assumption is not necessary for a valid test of the null hypothesis of no difference in population distributions but if it is not satisfied the interpretation of a statistically significant result is difficult.

Two samples

Unpaired case

Suppose $x_1, x_2, \ldots, x_{n_1}$ represent the n_1 observations in a sample from one population and $y_1, y_2, \ldots, y_{n_2}$ the n_2 observations on the same variable in a sample from a second population, where both sets of data are thought not to come from Normal distributions. The difference between the two population medians is estimated by the median of all the possible $n_1 \times n_2$ differences $x_i - y_j$ (for $i = 1$ to n_1 and $j = 1$ to n_2).

The confidence interval for the difference between the two population medians or means is also derived through these $n_1 \times n_2$ differences.[2] For an approximate $100(1 - \alpha)\%$ confidence interval first calculate

$$K = W_{\alpha/2} - \frac{n_1(n_1 + 1)}{2},$$

where $W_{\alpha/2}$ is the $100\alpha/2$ percentile of the distribution of the Mann–Whitney test statistic.[2] The Kth smallest to the Kth largest of the $n_1 \times n_2$ differences then determine the $100(1 - \alpha)\%$ confidence interval. Values of K for finding approximate 90%, 95%, and 99% confidence intervals ($\alpha = 0.10$, 0·05, and 0·01 respectively), together with the associated exact levels of confidence, for sample sizes of up to 25 are given directly in Table 18.5.

For studies where each sample size is greater than about 25, special tables are not required and K can be calculated approximately[2] as

$$K = \frac{n_1 n_2}{2} - \left(z_{1-\alpha/2} \times \sqrt{\frac{n_1 n_2(n_1 + n_2 + 1)}{12}} \right),$$

rounded up to the next integer value, where $z_{1-\alpha/2}$ is the appropriate value from the standard Normal distribution for the $100(1 - \alpha/2)$ percentile.

<hr>

Worked example

Consider the data in Table 5.1 on the globulin fraction of plasma (g/l) in two groups of 10 patients given by Swinscow.[6] The computations are made easier if the data in each group are first ranked into increasing order of magnitude and then all the group 1 minus group 2 differences

Table 5.1 Globulin fraction of plasma (g/l) in two groups of 10 patients[6]

Group 1	38	26	29	41	36	31	32	30	35	33
Group 2	45	28	27	38	40	42	39	39	34	45

Table 5.2 Differences in globulin fraction of plasma (g/l) between individuals in two groups of 10 patients[6]

Group 2	Group 1									
	26	29	30	31	32	33	35	36	38	41
27	−1	2	3	4	5	6	8	9	11	14
28	−2	1	2	3	4	5	7	8	10	13
34	−8	−5	−4	−3	−2	−1	1	2	4	7
38	−12	−9	−8	−7	−6	−5	−3	−2	0	3
39	−13	−10	−9	−8	−7	−6	−4	−3	−1	2
39	−13	−10	−9	−8	−7	−6	−4	−3	−1	2
40	−14	−11	−10	−9	−8	−7	−5	−4	−2	1
42	−16	−13	−12	−11	−10	−9	−7	−6	−4	−1
45	−19	−16	−15	−14	−13	−12	−10	−9	−7	−4
45	−19	−16	−15	−14	−13	−12	−10	−9	−7	−4

calculated as in Table 5.2. The estimate of the difference in population medians is now given by the median of these differences.

From the 100 differences in Table 5.2 the 50th smallest difference is −6 g/l and the 51st is −5 g/l, so the median difference is estimated as $[-6 + (-5)]/2 = -5.5$ g/l.

To calculate an approximate 95% confidence interval for the difference in population medians the value of $K = 24$ is found for $n_1 = 10$, $n_2 = 10$, and $\alpha = 0.05$ from Table 18.5. The 24th smallest difference is −10 g/l and the 24th largest is +1 g/l. The approximate 95% confidence interval (exact level 95·7%) for the difference in population medians or means is thus from −10 g/l to +1 g/l.

Paired case

Paired cases include, for example, studies of repeated measurements of the same variable on the same individuals over time and matched case-control comparisons. In these cases the paired differences are the observations of main interest. The method for finding confidence intervals described here assumes that, as well as the two distributions being identical except in location, the distribution of the paired differences is symmetrical. If this additional assumption seems unreasonable then the method described previously for a single sample can be applied to the paired differences.

Suppose that in a sample of size n the differences for each matched pair of measurements are $d_1, d_2, \ldots, d_n$. The difference between the two population medians is estimated by calculating all the $n(n + 1)/2$ possible averages of two of these differences taken together, including each difference with itself, and selecting their median.

The confidence interval for the difference between the population medians is also derived using these averaged differences. For an approximate $100(1-\alpha)\%$ confidence interval first find the value of $W_{\alpha/2}$ as the $100\alpha/2$ percentile of the distribution of the Wilcoxon one sample test statistic.[2] Then if $W_{\alpha/2} = K^*$, then the K^*th smallest to the K^*th largest of the averaged differences determine the $100(1-\alpha)\%$ confidence interval. Values of K^* for finding approximate 90%, 95%, and 99% confidence intervals ($\alpha = 0.10$, 0.05, and 0.01), together with the associated exact levels of confidence, are given directly for sample sizes of up to 50 in Table 18.6. In general the coverage probability is only slightly higher than the specified one.

For sample sizes of about 50 or more, special tables are not required and K^* can be calculated approximately[2] as

$$K^* = \frac{n(n+1)}{4} - \left(z_{1-\alpha/2} \times \sqrt{\frac{n(n+1)(2n+1)}{24}} \right),$$

rounded up to the next integer value, where $z_{1-\alpha/2}$ is the appropriate value from the standard Normal distribution for the $100(1-\alpha/2)$ percentile.

Worked example

Consider further the β-endorphin concentrations in subjects running in a half marathon where 11 people were studied both before and after the event.[5] The before and after concentrations (pmol/l) and their differences ordered by increasing size were as given in Table 5.3.

All the possible $n(n+1)/2$ averages in this case where $n = 11$ give the 66 averages shown in Table 5.4. Thus, having found $K^* = 11$ for $n = 11$ and

Table 5.3 β-endorphin concentrations in 11 runners before and after a half marathon[5]

Subject number	Before	After	After − before
1	10·6	14·6	4·0
2	5·2	15·6	10·4
3	8·4	20·2	11·8
4	9·0	20·9	11·9
5	6·6	24·0	17·4
6	4·6	25·0	20·4
7	14·1	35·2	21·1
8	5·2	30·2	25·0
9	4·4	30·0	25·6
10	17·4	46·2	28·8
11	7·2	37·0	29·8

Table 5.4 Averages of differences in β-endorphin concentrations in 11 runners before and after a half marathon.[5]

					Change						
Change	4·0	10·4	11·8	11·9	17·4	20·4	21·1	25·0	25·6	28·8	29·8
4·0	4·00	7·20	7·90	7·95	10·70	12·20	12·55	14·50	14·80	16·40	16·90
10·4		10·40	11·10	11·15	13·90	15·40	15·75	17·70	18·00	19·60	20·10
11·8			11·80	11·85	14·60	16·10	16·45	18·40	18·70	20·30	20·80
11·9				11·90	14·65	16·15	16·50	18·45	18·75	20·35	20·85
17·4					17·40	18·90	19·25	21·20	21·50	23·10	23·60
20·4						20·40	20·75	22·70	23·00	24·60	25·10
21·1							21·10	23·05	23·35	24·95	25·45
25·0								25·00	25·30	26·90	27·40
25·6									25·60	27·20	27·70
28·8										28·80	29·30
29·8											29·80

$\alpha = 0.05$ from Table 18.6, the 11 smallest averages are 4·00, 7·20, 7·90, 7·95, 10·40, 10·70, 11·10, 11·15, 11·80, 11·85, and 11·90; and the 11 largest averages are 25·10, 25·30, 25·45, 25·60, 26·90, 27·20, 27·40, 27·70, 28·80, 29·30, and 29·80. The approximate 95% (exact 95·8%) confidence interval for the difference between the population medians or means is thus given as 11·9 to 25·1 pmol/l around the sample median which is 18·8 pmol/l (the average of the 33rd and 34th ranked observations, 18·75 and 18·90, in the table of average differences). The triangular table of average differences helps to identify the required values, but a computer package such as MINITAB[3] can rank the averages in order and select the appropriate ranked values.

Comment

The methods summarised above for the confidence intervals for differences between two medians can be applied to the difference between two means. However, this method would only be used when the means involved arise from a symmetric distribution which is not Normal such as a rectangular distribution.

A method for calculating confidence intervals for Spearman's rank correlation coefficient, the non-parametric equivalent of the product moment correlation coefficient, is given in chapter 8.

Technical note

It should be noted that there are differences of presentation in the tables referred to in Conover,[2] *Geigy scientific tables*,[7] and elsewhere.

These result from the discrete nature of the distributions and whether[7] or not[2] the tabulated values are part of the critical region for the test of the null hypothesis. MINITAB[3] uses large sample formulae with continuity corrections for computing the coverage probabilities of the confidence intervals for differences between medians even for sample sizes less than 20. This can lead to inaccuracies in the coverage probabilities given by the program. Alternative methods for calculating confidence intervals for medians, and differences in medians, based on the 'bootstrap' are given in chapter 13.

1 Bland M. *An introduction to medical statistics*. 2nd edn. Oxford: Oxford University Press, 1995: 89–92, 165–6.
2 Conover WJ. *Practical non-parametric statistics*. 2nd edn. New York: John Wiley, 1980: table A3, 223–5, table A7, 288–90, table A13.
3 Ryan BF, Joiner BL, Rogosa D. *Minitab handbook*. 3rd edn. Boston: Duxbury Press, 1994.
4 Hill ID. 95% confidence limits for the median. *J Statist Comput Simulation* 1987;**28**:80–1.
5 Dale G, Fleetwood JA, Weddell A, Ellis RD, Sainsbury JRC. β-Endorphin: a factor in "fun run" collapse. *BMJ* 1987;**294**:1004.
6 Swinscow TDV. *Statistics at square one*. 9th edn. (Revised by MJ Campbell). London: BMJ Publishing Group, 1996: 92–9.
7 Lentner C, ed. *Geigy scientific tables*. Volume 2. 8th edn. Basle: Ciba-Geigy, 1982: 156–62, 163.

6 Proportions and their differences

ROBERT G NEWCOMBE,
DOUGLAS G ALTMAN

Proportions are used to summarise data for binary variables, that is, variables that can take two possible values, such as presence or absence of a symptom, success or failure of a treatment. In this chapter we present methods for constructing confidence intervals for single proportions and for differences between two proportions.

We describe two sets of methods. The traditional methods are based on the standard approach (see chapter 3) of taking a multiple of the standard error either side of the estimated quantity, here either the sample proportion or difference between two proportions. These methods are very widely used, and were the only ones given in the first edition of this book. Although they perform quite well in many cases, they have certain deficiencies, and are not valid when zeros or small numbers are involved.[1-3] Alternative methods[2-4] are now available that perform much better irrespective of the numbers involved. These methods are not as simple or intuitive, but give much better results across all circumstances. We refer to them below as 'recommended' methods.

Worked examples are given to illustrate each method. The calculations have been carried out to full arithmetic precision, as is recommended practice, but intermediate steps are shown as rounded results. In each case, both the calculated lower and upper limits are often expressed as percentages by multiplying by 100.

Confidence intervals convey only the effects of sampling variation on the estimated proportions and their differences and cannot control for other non-sampling errors such as biases in study design, conduct, or analysis (see chapter 3).

Single sample

Traditional method

If r is the observed number of subjects with some feature in a sample of size n then the estimated proportion who have the feature is $p = r/n$. The proportion who do not have the feature is $q = 1 - p$. The standard error of p is $\mathrm{SE}(p) = \sqrt{pq/n}$. Using the general approach of chapter 3, the $100(1 - \alpha)\%$ confidence interval for the proportion in the population is calculated as

$$p - [z_{1 - \alpha/2} \times \mathrm{SE}(p)] \quad \text{to} \quad p + [z_{1 - \alpha/2} \times \mathrm{SE}(p)]$$

where $z_{1 - \alpha/2}$ is the $100(1 - \alpha/2)$ percentile from the standard Normal distribution. Values of $z_{1 - \alpha/2}$ can be found from Table 18.1. Thus, for a 95% confidence interval $z_{1 - \alpha/2} = 1\cdot96$; this value does not depend on the sample size, as it does for the t distribution (chapter 4).

This traditional method is adequate in many circumstances, but it is based on an approximation. It should not be used for very low observed proportions, such as the prevalence of a disease, or very high ones, such as the sensitivity or specificity of a good diagnostic test (see chapter 10). The restriction on the use of the traditional method is usually given as a requirement that neither r nor $n - r$ is less than 5. Failure to observe this restriction leads to anomalies of several kinds.[1] Although the objective is to achieve a pre-stated probability, usually 95%, including the population proportion, in practice the attained coverage probability is much lower. The calculated limits lead to too extreme an interpretation of the data, and sometimes do not make sense. These problems are illustrated below.

In such cases an 'exact' but more complex method of calculating confidence intervals for population proportions is often used (see chapter 13 for an explanation of the term 'exact'). Exact values for 95% and 99% confidence intervals for $n = 2$ to 100 are given in *Geigy scientific tables*.[5] The direct calculation described below is arguably[6] better, in terms of closeness of the achieved coverage probability to its nominal value (95%, 99%, etc.). There is also some advantage in having a single method which can be applied in all cases.

Recommended method

The recommended method[4] has better statistical properties than the traditional method. First, calculate the three quantities

$$A = 2r + z^2; \quad B = z\sqrt{z^2 + 4rq}; \quad \text{and} \quad C = 2(n + z^2),$$

where z is as before the appropriate value, that is $z_{1-\alpha/2}$, from the standard Normal distribution. Then the confidence interval for the population proportion is given by

$$(A - B)/C \quad \text{to} \quad (A + B)/C.$$

This method has the considerable advantage that it can be used for any data. When there are no observed events, r and hence p are both zero, and the recommended confidence interval simplifies to 0 to $z^2/(n + z^2)$. When $r = n$ so that $p = 1$, the interval becomes $n/(n + z^2)$ to 1. This case is discussed in more detail later.

Worked example: large numbers

Out of 263 patients giving their views on the use of personal computers in general practice, 81 thought that the privacy of their medical file had been reduced.[7] Thus $p = 81/263 = 0.308$ and the standard error of p is

$$\text{SE}(p) = \sqrt{\frac{0.308 \times (1 - 0.308)}{263}} = 0.0285.$$

The 95% confidence interval for the population value of the proportion of patients thinking their privacy was reduced is then given as

$$0.308 - (1.96 \times 0.0285) \quad \text{to} \quad 0.308 + (1.96 \times 0.0285)$$

that is, from 0.252 to 0.364.

The recommended method gives a very similar interval, from 0.255 to 0.366.

Worked example: small numbers

A strength of the new method is that it can be used even when the observed proportion is very small (or very large), in situations where the traditional method is not valid. Of 29 female prisoners who did not inject drugs, 1 was found to be positive on testing for HIV on discharge.[8] Here $p = 1/29 = 0.034$ and $q = 0.966$. We calculate $A = 2 \times 1 + 1.96^2 = 5.84$, $B = 1.96 \times \sqrt{(1.96^2 + 4 \times 1 \times 0.966)} = 5.44$, and $C = 2 \times (29 + 1.96^2) = 65.68$. Then the 95% confidence interval for the prevalence of HIV positivity in the population of such women is given by $(5.84 - 5.44)/65.68 = 0.006$ to $(5.84 + 5.44)/65.68 = 0.172$, that is, from 0.6% to 17%.

In the same study,[8] there were 20 homosexual or bisexual males, none of whom tested positive. The estimated prevalence for this case is 0, with 95% confidence interval from 0 to $1.96^2/(20 + 1.96^2) = 0.161$, that is, from 0 to 16%.

Note that the confidence interval is not symmetric around p unless $p = \frac{1}{2}$, by contrast to the traditional method. If we were to use the traditional method to calculate a 95% confidence interval for the proportion 1/29 considered above we would get -3% to 10% which includes impossible negative values. The problem is due to the interval being symmetric around the observed proportion of 3·4%. In fact, an observed proportion of 1 out of 29 would occur about as often if the population proportion was 17% as if it was 0·6%. This asymmetry may at first seem surprising, but applies more widely, to confidence intervals for differences between proportions (described below), to quantities such as relative risks and odds ratios (chapter 7) and in non-parametric analyses (chapter 5).

Conversely, the traditional method fails to produce an interval for a zero proportion such as 0/20, we would obtain 0 for the upper limit as well as the lower one. This is inappropriate because the true population prevalence could well be large—especially in this example. The traditional method yields a zero width confidence interval irrespective of the sample size or the nominal coverage (95%, 99%, etc.). Similar problems occur when p is at or near 1.

Two samples: unpaired case

The difference between two population proportions is estimated by $D = p_1 - p_2$, the difference between the observed proportions in the two samples. It does not matter which proportion is taken as p_1, and which as p_2, so long as consistent usage is maintained.

Traditional method

The confidence interval for the difference between two population proportions is constructed round $p_1 - p_2$, the difference between the observed proportions in the two samples of sizes n_1 and n_2. The standard error of $p_1 - p_2$ is

$$\text{SE}(D) = \sqrt{\frac{p_1(1 - p_1)}{n_1} + \frac{p_2(1 - p_2)}{n_2}}.$$

The confidence interval for the population difference in proportions is then given by

$$D - z_{1-\alpha/2} \times \text{SE}(D) \quad \text{to} \quad D + z_{1-\alpha/2} \times \text{SE}(D),$$

where $z_{1-\alpha/2}$ is found as for the single sample case.

Negative values are reasonable for any difference between two proportions, which can meaningfully take any value between -1

and +1. Nonetheless the same restrictions on validity apply as for the single sample. The traditional method should thus not be used for small samples although it is hard to specify precisely the range of validity. It may be an unsafe approach with fewer than 30 in each group or if the observed proportions are outside the range 0·1 to 0·9.

Recommended method

The recommended method can again be used for any data. Calculate l_1 and u_1, the lower and upper limits that define the $100(1 - \alpha)\%$ confidence interval for the first sample, and l_2 and u_2, the lower and upper limits for the second sample, using the recommended method in the previous section. Then the $100(1 - \alpha)\%$ confidence interval for the population difference in proportions is calculated as

$$D - \sqrt{(p_1 - l_1)^2 + (u_2 - p_2)^2} \quad \text{to} \quad D + \sqrt{(p_2 - l_2)^2 + (u_1 - p_1)^2}$$

(this being method 10 of Newcombe[2]). Note that, just as for the single sample case, D is not generally at the midpoint of the interval.

Worked example: large numbers

A collaborative clinical trial[9] assessed the value of extracorporeal membrane oxygenation for term neonates with severe respiratory failure. 63 of the 93 patients randomised to active treatment survived to one year compared with 38 of the 92 infants who received conventional management. Thus, $p_1 = 63/93 = 0.677$ and $p_2 = 38/92 = 0.413$. The difference between these two proportions is estimated as $0.677 - 0.413 = 0.264$. The standard error of the difference is

$$\sqrt{\frac{0.677 \times (1 - 0.677)}{93} + \frac{0.413 \times (1 - 0.413)}{92}} = 0.071.$$

Using the traditional method, the 95% confidence interval for the difference between the two population proportions is then $0.264 - 1.96 \times 0.071$ to $0.264 + 1.96 \times 0.071$, that is, from 0.126 to 0.403. In this case the recommended method gives a very similar interval, from 0.121 to 0.393.

Worked example: small numbers

Goodfield et al.[10] reported adverse effects in 85 patients receiving either terbinafine or placebo treatment for dermatophyte onchomyosis; the results are shown in Table 6.1. Here, the proportions experiencing

49

Table 6.1 Numbers of patients experiencing respiratory problems in patients receiving either terbinafine or placebo[10]

| | Treatment group | |
Response	Terbinafine (Group 1)	Placebo (Group 2)
Respiratory problems	5	0
No respiratory problems	51	29
Total	56	29

respiratory problems were $p_1 = 5/56 = 0.089$ and $p_2 = 0/29 = 0.0$ for active and placebo groups respectively, suggesting that an extra 9% of patients would experience respiratory problems if given terbinafine rather than placebo.

Using the recommended method described above for the single proportion, 95% confidence intervals for these proportions are 0.039 to 0.193 and 0 to 0.117 respectively. The 95% confidence interval for the difference between the two population proportions is then given by

$$(0.089 - 0) - \sqrt{(0.089 - 0.039)^2 + (0.117 - 0)^2} \quad \text{to}$$

$$(0.089 - 0) + \sqrt{(0 - 0)^2 + (0.193 - 0.089)^2}$$

that is, from -0.038 to $+0.193$. Thus, although the best estimate of the difference in proportions experiencing respiratory problems is 9%, the 95% confidence interval ranges from -4% (indicating 4% fewer problems on the active treatment) to $+19\%$ (indicating 19% more problems on the active treatment), showing the imprecision due to the limited sample size.

Two samples: paired case

Examples of paired binary data, to be summarised by presenting and comparing proportions, include the following:

(a) Forty-one subjects were classified[11] by a clinical investigator and by a laboratory test which is regarded as definitive. The laboratory test classified 14 subjects as positive. The investigator classified as positive all 14 of these and also 5 of the subjects who subsequently proved test negative.

(b) In an individually paired case-control study,[12] 23 out of 35 cases, but only 13 out of 35 matched controls, were positive for exposure to the risk factor under study.

(c) In a crossover trial[13] comparing home and hospital physiotherapy for chronic multiple sclerosis, 31 out of 40 patients

Table 6.2 Classification of subjects undergoing a thallium-201 stress test as normal or ischaemic by clinical investigator and core laboratory[11]

| | Core laboratory | | |
Clinical investigator	Ischaemic	Normal	Total
Ischaemic	$r = 14$	$s = 5$	19
Normal	$t = 0$	$u = 22$	22
Total	14	27	$n = 41$

gave a positive response to treatment at home, whereas 25 patients gave a positive response to treatment in hospital.

(d) Respiratory symptom questionnaires were administered[14,15] to a cohort of 1319 children at age 12 and again at age 14. At age 12 356 children (27%) were reported to have had severe colds in the past 12 months compared to 468 (35%) at age 14.

The data may be presented in the same way in each situation, but with labelling to correspond to the context. Either a standard 2×2 format may be used, as in Table 6.2, or a four-row table, as in Table 6.3.

Table 6.2 presents the data for example (a) and also shows the labelling of the frequencies used in this section. In examples (a), (c), and (d) above we characterise the strength of the effect by the difference between two proportions. In case (b), it is more relevant to characterise the strength of the association by using the odds ratio, as in chapter 7.

The proportions of subjects with the feature on the two occasions are $p_1 = (r + s)/n$ and $p_2 = (r + t)/n$, and the difference between them is $D = p_1 - p_2 = (s - t)/n$. Note that we cannot get the confidence interval for the difference from p_1 and p_2 (and n) alone—we need to know the four counts r, s, t and u.

Table 6.3 Proportions of children reporting severe colds within the past 12 months, at ages 12 and 14[14,15]

Severe colds at age 12	Severe colds at age 14	Number of children
Yes	Yes	212
Yes	No	144
No	Yes	256
No	No	707
Total		1319

51

Traditional method

The standard error of the difference between the two proportions is

$$SE(D) = \frac{1}{n} \times \sqrt{s + t - \frac{(s-t)^2}{n}}.$$

The $100(1-\alpha)\%$ confidence interval for the population difference between proportions is then given as

$$D - z_{1-\alpha/2} \times SE(D) \quad \text{to} \quad D + z_{1-\alpha/2} \times SE(D),$$

where $z_{1-\alpha/2}$ is found as for the single sample case. An exact method is available and is sometimes used when the numbers in the study are small. The approach is similar to that described in chapter 7 to find the confidence interval for the odds ratio in a matched case-control study. We do not describe it here as the recommended approach described below obviates the need to use it and is greatly superior.

Recommended method

First (as for the unpaired case) calculate separate $100(1-\alpha)\%$ confidence intervals for p_1 and p_2, using the recommended method, as l_1 to u_1 and l_2 to u_2. Next, a quantity ϕ is calculated, which is used to correct for the fact that p_1 and p_2 are not independent: it is a kind of correlation coefficient (see chapter 8) for the binary case, and is closely related to the familiar chi squared (χ^2) test. It is usually positive, and thus reduces the interval width. If any of the quantities $r+s$, $t+u$, $r+t$ or $s+u$ is zero, then $\phi = 0$. Otherwise, calculate $A = (r+s)(t+u)(r+t)(s+u)$ and $B = ru - st$. Then obtain C as follows:

$C = B - n/2$ if B is greater than $n/2$ ($B > n/2$);

$C = 0$ if B is between 0 and $n/2$ ($0 \le B \le n/2$);

$C = B$ if B is less than 0 ($B < 0$).

Then calculate $\phi = C/\sqrt{A}$.

The $100(1-\alpha)\%$ confidence interval for the population value of the difference between these proportions (D) is then

$$D - \sqrt{(p_1 - l_1)^2 - 2\phi(p_1 - l_1)(u_2 - p_2) + (u_2 - p_2)^2} \quad \text{to}$$

$$D + \sqrt{(p_2 - l_2)^2 - 2\phi(p_2 - l_2)(u_1 - p_1) + (u_1 - p_1)^2}.$$

(This is method 10 of Newcombe.[3])

Worked example: large numbers

1319 children were asked at age 12 and again at age 14 about respiratory illnesses in the preceding 12 months.[14,15] The paired data summarising numbers reporting severe colds are given in Table 6.3. We take p_1 to be the proportion with severe colds at age 14, that is $p_1 = 468/1319 = 0.355$, and p_2 to be the proportion at age 12, that is $p_2 = 356/1319 = 0.270$. The quantity of interest is the increase in the period prevalence, $D = p_1 - p_2 = 0.355 - 0.270 = 0.085$.

The standard error of the difference $D = p_1 - p_2$ is found from the formula given above as

$$SE(D) = \frac{1}{1319} \times \sqrt{144 + 256 - \frac{(144 - 256)^2}{1319}} = 0.015.$$

The 95% confidence interval for the difference between the two population proportions by the traditional method is then given by

$$0.085 - (1.96 \times 0.015) \quad \text{to} \quad 0.085 + (1.96 \times 0.015),$$

that is, from 0.056 to 0.114.

The recommended method gives an interval from 0.055 to 0.114 for D, which is very similar to the interval calculated by the traditional method.

Worked example: small numbers

In a reliability exercise carried out as part of the Multicenter Study of Silent Myocardial Ischemia,[11] 41 patients were randomly selected from those who had undergone a thallium-201 stress test. The 41 sets of images were classified as normal or not by the core thallium laboratory and, independently, by clinical investigators from different centres who had participated in training sessions intended to produce standardisation. Table 6.2 presents the results for one of the participating clinical investigators.

The proportions of subjects classified as positive both by the investigator and by the laboratory were $p_1 = 0.463$ and $p_2 = 0.341$ (19/41 and 14/41) respectively; the investigator thus overdiagnosed abnormality by $0.463 - 0.341 = 0.122$, that is in 12% more cases than the laboratory test. Here, 95% confidence intervals for p_1 and p_2 are 0.321 to 0.613 and 0.216 to 0.494 respectively. We calculate

$$A = (14 + 5) \times (0 + 22) \times (14 + 0) \times (5 + 22) = 158\,004,$$

$$B = 14 \times 22 - 5 \times 0 = 308,$$

since $B > n/2, \quad C = B - n/2 = 308 - 41/2 = 287.5,$

$$\phi = 287.5/\sqrt{158\,004} = 0.723.$$

The lower limit of the required 95% confidence interval is then

$$0\cdot122 - \sqrt{\begin{array}{l}(0\cdot463 - 0\cdot321)^2 - 2 \times 0\cdot723 \times (0\cdot463 - 0\cdot321) \times \\ (0\cdot494 - 0\cdot341) + (0\cdot494 - 0\cdot341)^2\end{array}}$$

$$= 0\cdot122 - 0\cdot110 = 0\cdot011.$$

The upper limit is

$$0\cdot122 + \sqrt{\begin{array}{l}(0\cdot341 - 0\cdot216)^2 - 2 \times 0\cdot723 \times (0\cdot341 - 0\cdot216) \times \\ (0\cdot613 - 0\cdot463) + (0\cdot613 - 0\cdot463)^2\end{array}}$$

$$= 0\cdot122 + 0\cdot105 = 0\cdot226.$$

The 95% confidence interval for the population difference in proportions is 0·011 to 0·226, or approximately +1% to +23%.

When no events are observed

Given that in a sample of individuals no cases are observed with the outcome of interest, what can be said about the true prevalence in the population?

Many authors have noted that the 95% confidence interval for an observed proportion of zero in a sample of size n has upper limit approximately $3/n$ whatever the value of n.[16,17] The value is a little less than 3 for small samples, but this 'rule of three' is a reliable guide for samples of more than 50. The value of 3 is, however, the upper limit of a one-sided confidence interval.[5] For comparability with the standard two-sided intervals it is necessary to take a one-sided 97·5% confidence interval, for which the upper limit is $3\cdot7/n$.

These calculations are not based on the traditional method to derive confidence intervals but the exact method referred to earlier, which is sometimes known as the Clopper–Pearson method.[5] A strength of the recommended method given earlier is that it can safely be used in this extreme situation. The upper limit of the confidence interval when there are no observed events becomes $z^2/(n + z^2)$, where z is the appropriate value from the Normal distribution. For a 95% confidence interval $z = 1\cdot96$, so that the 95% confidence interval for an observed proportion of 0 is from 0 to $3\cdot84/(n + 3\cdot84)$. For a 99% confidence interval $z = 2\cdot576$, and the upper limit is $6\cdot64/(n + 6\cdot64)$.

If an easily memorable formula is wanted we suggest a new 'rule of four' in which the upper limit of the 95% confidence interval is $4/(n + 4)$, which is a close approximation to the correct value.

The same principles apply equally to the case where the event is observed in all individuals. Here the confidence interval for the population proportion is from $n/(n + z^2)$ to 1.

Software

Both the traditional and recommended methods are included in the CIA software accompanying this book. The recommended methods are referred to as Wilson's method for the single sample case and Newcombe's method for the comparisons of two proportions (paired or unpaired).

Technical note

Although for quantitative data and means there is a direct correspondence between the confidence interval approach and a t test of the null hypothesis at the associated level of statistical significance, this is not exactly so for qualitative data and proportions. The lack of direct correspondence is small and should not result in changes of interpretation.

1 Newcombe RG. Two-sided confidence intervals for the single proportion: comparison of seven methods. *Stat Med* 1998;**17**:857–72.
2 Newcombe RG. Interval estimation for the difference between independent proportions: comparison of eleven methods. *Stat Med* 1998;**17**:873–90.
3 Newcombe RG. Improved confidence intervals for the difference between binomial proportions based on paired data. *Stat Med* 1998; **17**:2635–50.
4 Wilson EB. Probable inference, the law of succession, and statistical inference. *J Am Stat Assoc* 1927;**22**:209–12.
5 Lentner C, ed. *Geigy scientific tables*. Volume 2. 8th edn. Basle: Geigy, 1982: 89–102 and 186.
6 Agresti A, Coull BA. Approximate is better than "exact" for interval estimation of binomial proportions. *Am Stat* 1998;**52**:119–26.
7 Rethans J-J, Hoppener P, Wolfs G, Diederiks J. Do personal computers make doctors less personal? *BMJ* 1988;**296**:1446–8.
8 Turnbull PJ, Stimson GV, Dolan KA. Prevalence of HIV infection among ex-prisoners in England. *BMJ* 1992;**304**:90–1.
9 Roberts TE. Extracorporeal Membrane Oxygenation Economics Working Group. Economic evaluation and randomised controlled trial of extracorporeal membrane oxygenation: UK collaborative trial. *BMJ* 1998;**317**:911–16.
10 Goodfield MJD, Andrew L, Evans EGV. Short-term treatment of dermatophyte onchomyosis with terbinafine. *BMJ* 1992;**304**:1151–4.
11 Bigger JT and the MSSMI investigators. Longitudinal (natural history) studies of silent myocardial ischemia. In Morganroth JJ, Moore EN (eds). *Silent myocardial ischemia*. Boston: Martinus Nijhoff, 1988.
12 Eason J, Markowe HLJ. Controlled investigation of deaths from asthma in hospitals in the North East Thames region. *BMJ* 1987;**294**:1255–8.
13 Wiles CM, Newcombe RG, Fuller KJ, Shaw S, Furnival-Doran JF, Pickersgill TP, Morgan A. A controlled randomised crossover trial of the effects of physiotherapy on mobility in chronic multiple sclerosis. Submitted for publication.

14 Holland WW, Bailey P, Bland JM. Long-term consequences of respiratory disease in infancy. *J Epidemiol Comm Hlth* 1978;**32**:256–9.
15 Bland M. *An introduction to medical statistics.* 2nd ed. Oxford: Oxford Medical Publications, 1995: 241–3.
16 Rümke CL. Implications of the statement: no side effects were observed. *N Engl J Med* 1975;**292**:372–3.
17 Hanley JA, Lippman-Hand A. If nothing goes wrong, is everything all right? Interpreting zero numerators. *JAMA* 1983;**249**:1743–5.

7 Epidemiological studies

JULIE A MORRIS, MARTIN J GARDNER

The techniques for obtaining confidence intervals for estimates of relative risks, attributable risks and odds ratios are described. These can come either from an incidence study, where, for example, the frequency of a congenital malformation at birth is compared in two defined groups of mothers, or from a case-control study, where a group of patients with the disease of interest (the cases) is compared with another group of people without the disease (the controls).

The methods of obtaining confidence intervals for standardised disease ratios and rates in studies of incidence, prevalence, and mortality are described. Such rates and ratios are commonly calculated to enable appropriate comparisons to be made between study groups after adjustment for confounding factors like age and sex. The most frequently used standardised indices are the standardised incidence ratio (SIR) and the standardised mortality ratio (SMR).

Some of the methods given here are large sample approximations but will give reasonable estimates for small studies. Appropriate design principles for these types of study have to be adhered to, since confidence intervals convey only the effects of sampling variation on the precision of the estimated statistics. They cannot control for other errors such as biases due to the selection of inappropriate controls or in the methods of collecting the data.

Relative risks, attributable risks and odds ratios

Incidence study

Suppose that the incidence or frequency of some outcome is assessed in two groups of individuals defined by the presence or

Table 7.1 Classification of outcome by group characteristic

Outcome	Group characteristic	
	Present	Absent
Yes	A	B
No	C	D
Total	$A + C$	$B + D$

absence of some characteristic. The data from such a study can be presented as in Table 7.1.

The outcome probabilities in exposed and unexposed individuals are estimated from the study groups by $A/(A + C)$ and $B/(B + D)$ respectively. An estimate, R, of the relative risk (or risk ratio) from exposure is given by the ratio of these proportions, so that

$$R = \frac{A/(A + C)}{B/(B + D)}.$$

Confidence intervals for the population value of R can be constructed through a logarithmic transformation.[1] The standard error of $\log_e R$ is

$$\text{SE}(\log_e R) = \sqrt{\frac{C}{A(A + C)} + \frac{B}{B(B + D)}}.$$

This can also be written as

$$\text{SE}(\log_e R) = \sqrt{\frac{1}{A} - \frac{1}{A + C} + \frac{1}{B} - \frac{1}{B + D}}.$$

A $100(1 - \alpha)\%$ confidence interval for R is found by first calculating the two quantities

$$W = \log_e R - [z_{1 - \alpha/2} \times \text{SE}(\log_e R)]$$

and

$$X = \log_e R + [z_{1 - \alpha/2} \times \text{SE}(\log_e R)],$$

where $z_{1 - \alpha/2}$ is the appropriate value from the standard Normal distribution for the $100(1 - \alpha/2)$ percentile found in Table 18.1. The confidence interval for the population value of R is then given by exponentiating W and X as

$$e^W \quad \text{to} \quad e^X.$$

Table 7.2 Prevalence of *Helicobacter pylori* infection in preschool children according to mother's history of ulcer[2]

Infected with *H. pylori*	History of ulcer in mother	
	Yes	No
Yes	6	112
No	16	729
Total	22	841

Worked example

Brenner *et al.* reported the prevalence of *Helicobacter pylori* infection in preschool children according to parental history of duodenal or gastric ulcer.[2] The results are shown in Table 7.2.

An estimate of the relative risk of *Helicobacter pylori* infection associated with a history of ulcer in the mother is

$$R = \frac{6/22}{112/841} = 2 \cdot 05.$$

The standard error of $\log_e R$ is

$$\sqrt{\frac{1}{6} - \frac{1}{22} + \frac{1}{112} - \frac{1}{841}} = 0 \cdot 3591$$

from which for a 95% confidence interval

$$W = \log_e 2 \cdot 05 - (1 \cdot 96 \times 0 \cdot 3591) = 0 \cdot 0130$$

and

$$X = \log_e 2 \cdot 05 + (1 \cdot 96 \times 0 \cdot 3591) = 1 \cdot 4206.$$

The 95% confidence interval for the population value of R is then given as

$$e^{0 \cdot 0130} \quad \text{to} \quad e^{1 \cdot 4206}$$

that is, from 1·01 to 4·14. The estimated risk of *Helicobacter pylori* infection in children with a history of ulcer in the mother is 205% of that in children without a history of ulcer in the mother with a 95% confidence interval of 101% to 414%.

A measure of the proportion of individuals in the total population with the disease attributed to exposure to the risk factor is given by the attributable risk (AR). If p is the prevalence of the risk factor in the population and R is the relative risk for disease associated with the risk factor, then

$$AR = \frac{p(R - 1)}{1 + p(R - 1)}.$$

If the prevalence, p, is assumed to have negligible sampling variation, then the $100(1 - \alpha)\%$ confidence interval for AR can be derived by obtaining confidence limits for the relative risk, R, as described previously and substituting these into the formula for AR given above.[3] (See chapter 13 for discussion of this 'substitution' method.) This approach will give a reasonable approximation to confidence intervals derived from a more exact method. It is important to note that this method is not appropriate for substitution of a confounder-adjusted relative risk.[4,5]

Denoting the confidence interval for R by R_L to R_U, the $100(1 - \alpha)\%$ confidence interval for AR is given by

$$\frac{p(R_L - 1)}{1 + p(R_L - 1)} \quad \text{to} \quad \frac{p(R_U - 1)}{1 + p(R_U - 1)}.$$

Worked example

In the previous example, the prevalence of history of ulcer in mothers of preschool children is $22/863 = 0.0255$, and the relative risk of *Helicobacter pylori* infection associated with a history of ulcer is 2.05.[2] An estimate of the attributable risk is

$$AR = \frac{0.0255(2.05 - 1)}{1 + 0.0255(2.05 - 1)} = 0.0260.$$

As already calculated, the 95% confidence interval for R is given by $R_L = 1.01$ to $R_U = 4.14$. The 95% confidence interval for AR is thus

$$\frac{0.0255(1.01 - 1)}{1 + 0.0255(1.01 - 1)} \quad \text{to} \quad \frac{0.0255(4.14 - 1)}{1 + 0.0255(4.14 - 1)}$$

that is, from 0.0003 to 0.0741. The proportion of children with *Helicobacter pylori* infection due to history of ulcer in the mother is estimated at 26 per 1000 with a wide 95% confidence interval ranging from 0.3 per 1000 to 74 per 1000.

Unmatched case-control study

Suppose that groups of cases and controls are studied to assess exposure to a suspected causal factor. The data can be presented as in Table 7.3.

An approximate estimate of the relative risk for the disease associated with exposure to the factor can be obtained from a case-control study through the odds ratio,[6] the relative risk itself not being directly estimable with this study design. The odds ratio (OR) is given as

$$OR = \frac{ad}{bc}.$$

Table 7.3 Classification of exposure among cases and controls

Study group	Exposed Yes	Exposed No	Total
Cases	a	b	$a+b$
Controls	c	d	$c+d$
Total	$a+c$	$b+d$	n

A confidence interval for the population odds ratio can be constructed using several methods which vary in their ease and accuracy. The method described here (sometimes called the logit method) was devised by Woolf[7] and is widely recommended as a satisfactory approximation. The exception to this is when any of the numbers a, b, c, or d is small, when a more accurate but complex procedure should be used if suitable computer facilities are available. Further discussion and comparison of methods can be found in Breslow and Day.[8] The use of the following approach, however, should not in general lead to any misinterpretation of the results.

The logit method uses the Normal approximation to the distribution of the logarithm of the odds ratio ($\log_e OR$) in which the standard error is

$$\mathrm{SE}(\log_e OR) = \sqrt{\frac{1}{a} + \frac{1}{b} + \frac{1}{c} + \frac{1}{d}}.$$

A $100(1 - \alpha)\%$ confidence interval for OR is found by first calculating the two quantities

$$Y = \log_e OR - [z_{1-\alpha/2} \times \mathrm{SE}(\log_e OR)]$$

and

$$Z = \log_e OR + [z_{1-\alpha/2} \times \mathrm{SE}(\log_e OR)],$$

where $z_{1-\alpha/2}$ is the appropriate value from the standard Normal distribution for the $100(1 - \alpha/2)$ percentile (see Table 18.1). The confidence interval for the odds ratio in the population is then obtained by exponentiating Y and Z to give

$$e^Y \quad \text{to} \quad e^Z.$$

Worked example

ABO non-secretor state was determined for 114 patients with spondyloarthropathies and 334 controls[9] with the results shown in Table 7.4.

Table 7.4 ABO non-secretor state for 114 patients with spondyloarthropathies and 334 controls[9]

| | ABO non-secretor state | | |
Study group	Yes	No	Total
Cases	54	60	114
Controls	89	245	334
Total	143	305	448

The estimated odds ratio for spondyloarthropathies with ABO non-secretor state is $OR = (54 \times 245)/(60 \times 89) = 2{\cdot}48$. The standard error of $\log_e OR$ is

$$SE(\log_e OR) = \sqrt{\frac{1}{54} + \frac{1}{60} + \frac{1}{89} + \frac{1}{245}} = 0{\cdot}2247.$$

For a 95% confidence interval

$$Y = \log_e 2{\cdot}48 - (1{\cdot}96 \times 0{\cdot}2247) = 0{\cdot}4678$$

and

$$Z = \log_e 2{\cdot}48 + (1{\cdot}96 \times 0{\cdot}2247) = 1{\cdot}3487.$$

The 95% confidence interval for the population value of the odds ratio for spondyloarthropathies with ABO non-secretor state is then given as

$$e^{0{\cdot}4678} \quad \text{to} \quad e^{1{\cdot}3487}$$

that is, from $1{\cdot}59$ to $3{\cdot}85$. These results show that the estimated risk of spondyloarthropathy with ABO non-secretor state is 248% of that without ABO non-secretor state with 95% confidence interval of 159% to 385%.

More than two levels of exposure

If there are more than two levels of exposure, one can be chosen as a baseline with which each of the others is compared. Odds ratios and their associated confidence intervals are then calculated for each comparison in the same way as shown previously for only two levels of exposure.

A series of unmatched case-control studies

A combined estimate is sometimes required when independent estimates of the same odds ratio are available from each of K sets of data—for example, in a stratified analysis to control for confounding variables.

One approach is to use the logit method to give a pooled estimate of the odds ratio (OR_{logit}) and then derive a confidence interval for the odds ratio in a similar way to that for a single 2×2 table. The logit combined estimate (OR_{logit}) is defined by

$$\log_e OR_{\text{logit}} = \sum w_i \log_e OR_i \Big/ \sum w_i,$$

where $OR_i = a_i d_i / b_i c_i$ is the odds ratio in the ith table, a_i, b_i, c_i, and d_i are the frequencies in the ith 2×2 table, $n_i = a_i + b_i + c_i + d_i$, the summation $\sum$ is over $i = 1$ to K for the K tables and w_i is defined as

$$w_i = \frac{1}{(1/a_i) + (1/b_i) + (1/c_i) + (1/d_i)}.$$

The standard error of $\log_e (OR_{\text{logit}})$ is given by

$$SE(\log_e OR_{\text{logit}}) = \frac{1}{\sqrt{w}},$$

where $w = \sum w_i$.

A $100(1 - \alpha)\%$ confidence interval for OR_{logit} can then be found by calculating

$$U = \log_e OR_{\text{logit}} - [z_{1-\alpha/2} \times SE(\log_e OR_{\text{logit}})]$$

and

$$V = \log_e OR_{\text{logit}} + [z_{1-\alpha/2} \times SE(\log_e OR_{\text{logit}})]$$

where $z_{1-\alpha/2}$ is the appropriate value from the standard Normal distribution for the $100(1 - \alpha/2)$ percentile (see Table 18.1).

The confidence interval for the population value of OR_{logit} is given by exponentiating U and V as

$$e^U \quad \text{to} \quad e^V.$$

It is important to mention that, before combining independent estimates, there should be some reassurance that the separate odds ratios do not vary markedly, apart from sampling error.[6,8] Hence, a test for homogeneity of the odds ratio over the strata is recommended. Further discussion of homogeneity tests, methods for the calculation of 95% confidence intervals and a worked example are given in Breslow and Day.[8] The logit method is unsuitable if any of the numbers a_i, b_i, c_i, or d_i is small. This will happen, for example, with increasing stratification, and in such cases a more complex exact method is available.[8]

An alternative approach which gives a consistent estimate of the common odds ratio with large numbers of small strata is to use the Mantel–Haenszel pooled estimate of the odds ratio (OR_{M-H}) which is given by

$$OR_{M-H} = \sum \frac{a_i d_i}{n_i} \bigg/ \sum \frac{b_i c_i}{n_i}.$$

A method of calculating confidence intervals for this estimate is described in Armitage and Berry.[6] It is more complex, however, than the previous approach which extends the single case-control technique shown earlier. For samples of reasonable size both methods will usually give similar values for the combined odds ratio and confidence interval.

The scope of a stratified analysis for case-control studies can be extended using a logistic regression model.[8] This also enables the joint effects of two or more factors on disease risk to be assessed (see chapter 8).

Worked example

A number of studies examining the relationship of passive smoking exposure to lung cancer were reviewed by Wald et al.[10] The findings, which are shown in Table 7.5, included those from four studies of women in the USA. They are used below to illustrate the combination of results from independent sets of data. A test for homogeneity of the odds ratio provided no evidence of a difference between the four studies.

The logit combined estimate of the odds ratio (OR_{logit}) over the four studies is found to be 1·19. The standard error of $\log_e (OR_{logit})$ is 0·1694.

For a 95% confidence interval

$$U = \log_e 1·19 - (1·96 \times 0·1694) = -0·1581$$

and

$$V = \log_e 1·19 + (1·96 \times 0·1694) = 0·5060.$$

Table 7.5 Exposure to passive smoking among female lung cancer cases and controls in four studies[10]

	Lung cancer cases		Controls		
Study	Exposed (a)	Unexposed (b)	Exposed (c)	Unexposed (d)	Odds ratio
1	14	8	61	72	2·07
2	33	8	164	32	0·80
3	13	11	15	10	0·79
4	91	43	254	148	1·23

The 95% confidence interval for the population value of the odds ratio of lung cancer associated with passive smoking exposure is then given by

$$e^{-0.1581} \quad \text{to} \quad e^{0.5060}$$

that is, from 0·85 to 1·66. The risk of lung cancer with passive smoking exposure is estimated to be 119% of that with no passive smoking exposure with a 95% confidence interval of 85% to 166%.

If, alternatively, the Mantel–Haenszel method is used on these data the combined estimate of the odds ratio is found to be also 1·19, with a 95% confidence interval of 0·86 to 1·66, virtually the same result.

Matched case-control study

If each of n cases of a disease is matched to one control to form n pairs and each individual's exposure to a suspected causal factor is recorded the data can be presented as in Table 7.6. For this type of study an approximate estimate (in fact the Mantel–Haenszel estimate) of the relative risk of the disease associated with exposure is again given by the odds ratio which is now calculated as

$$OR = \frac{s}{t}.$$

An exact $100(1 - \alpha)$% confidence interval for the population value of OR is found by first determining a confidence interval for s (the number of case-control pairs with only the case exposed).[6] Conditional on the sum of the numbers of "discordant" pairs $(s + t)$ the number s can be considered as a Binomial variable with sample size $s + t$ and proportion $s/(s + t)$.

The $100(1 - \alpha)$% confidence interval for the population value of the Binomial proportion can be obtained from tables based on the Binomial distribution (for example, Lentner[11]). If this confidence interval is denoted by A_L to A_U the $100(1 - \alpha)$% confidence

Table 7.6 Classification of matched case-control pairs by exposure

| Exposure status | | |
Case	Control	Number of pairs
Yes	Yes	r
Yes	No	s
No	Yes	t
No	No	u
	Total	n

65

interval for the population value of OR is then given by

$$\frac{A_L}{1 - A_L} \quad \text{to} \quad \frac{A_U}{1 - A_U}.$$

Worked example

Thirty-five patients who died in hospital from asthma were individually matched for sex and age with 35 control subjects who had been discharged from the same hospital in the preceding year.[12] The inadequacy of monitoring of all patients while in hospital was independently assessed; the paired results are given in Table 7.7.

Table 7.7 Inadequacy of monitoring in hospital of deaths and survivors among 35 matched pairs of asthma patients[12]

Inadequacy of monitoring		Number of pairs
Deaths	Survivors	
Yes	Yes	10
Yes	No	13
No	Yes	3
No	No	9
	Total	35

The estimated odds ratio of dying in hospital associated with inadequate monitoring is $OR = 13/3 = 4.33$.

From the appropriate table for the Binomial distribution with sample size $s + t = 13 + 3 = 16$, proportion $s/(s + t) = 13/(13 + 3) = 0.81$, and $\alpha = 0.05$, the 95% confidence interval for the population value of the Binomial proportion is found to be $A_L = 0.5435$ to $A_U = 0.9595$. The 95% confidence interval for the population value of the odds ratio is thus

$$\frac{0.5435}{1 - 0.5435} \quad \text{to} \quad \frac{0.9595}{1 - 0.9595}$$

that is, from 1.19 to 23.69. The risk of dying in hospital following inadequate monitoring is estimated to be 433% of that with adequate monitoring, with a very wide 95% confidence interval ranging from 119% to 2369%, reflecting the imprecision in this estimate.

Matched case-control study with 1 : M matching

Sometimes each case is matched with more than one control. The odds ratio is then given by the Mantel–Haenszel estimate as

$$OR_{M-H} = \sum [(M - i + 1) \times n_{i-1}^{(1)}] \Big/ \sum (i \times n_i^{(0)}),$$

where M is the number of matched controls for each case, $n_{i-1}^{(1)}$ is the number of matched sets in which the case and $i-1$ of the matched controls are exposed, $n_i^{(0)}$ is the number of sets in which the case is unexposed and i of the matched controls are exposed, and the summation is from $i = 1$ to M.

A confidence interval for the population value of OR_{M-H} can be derived by one of the methods in Breslow and Day.[8] These authors also explain the calculation of a confidence interval for the odds ratio estimated from a study with a variable number of matched controls for each case.[8]

Incidence rates, standardised ratios and rates

Incidence rates

If x is the observed number of individuals with the outcome (or disease) of interest, and Py the number of person-years at risk, the incidence rate is given by $IR = x/Py$.

The $100(1 - \alpha)\%$ confidence interval for the population value of IR can be calculated by first assuming x to have a Poisson distribution, and finding its related confidence interval.[3] Table 18.3 gives 90%, 95% and 99% confidence intervals for x in the range 0 to 100. It also indicates how to obtain approximate confidence intervals for x taking values greater than 100. Denote this confidence interval by x_L to x_U. Assuming Py is a constant with no sampling variation, the $100(1 - \alpha)\%$ confidence interval for IR is given by

$$\frac{x_L}{Py} \quad \text{to} \quad \frac{x_U}{Py}.$$

Worked example

Nunn *et al.* published mortality figures for the period 1990–95 in a rural population in south-west Uganda.[13] They reported 28 deaths among children aged 5–12 years over 10 992 person-years of observation.

Taking $x = 28$ and $Py = 10\,992$, the death rate for 5–12-year olds is $IR = 28/10\,992 = 2.55$ deaths per 1000 person-years. The 95% confidence limits for the number of deaths, $x_L = 18.6$ and $x_U = 40.5$ are found from Table 18.3 with $x = 28$ and $\alpha = 0.05$.

The 95% confidence interval for the death rate is

$$\frac{18.6}{10\,992} \quad \text{to} \quad \frac{40.5}{10\,992}$$

that is, from 1.69 to 3.68 per 1000 person-years.

Standardised ratios

If O is the observed number of incident cases (or deaths) in a study group and E the expected number based on, for example, the age-specific disease incidence (or mortality) rates in a reference or standard population the standardised incidence ratio (SIR) or standardised mortality ratio (SMR) is O/E. This is usually called the indirect method of standardisation because the specific rates of a standard population are used in the calculation rather than the rates of the study population. The expected number is calculated as

$$E = \sum n_i DR_i,$$

where n_i is the number of individuals in age group i of the study group, DR_i is the death rate in age group i of the reference population, and $\sum$ denotes summation over all age groups.

The $100(1 - \alpha)\%$ confidence interval for the population value of O/E can be found by first regarding O as a Poisson variable and finding its related confidence interval[14] (see Table 18.3). Denote this confidence interval by O_L to O_U.

The $100(1 - \alpha)\%$ confidence interval for the population value of O/E is then given by

$$\frac{O_L}{E} \quad \text{to} \quad \frac{O_U}{E}.$$

Worked example

Roman *et al.* observed 64 cases of leukaemia in children under the age of 15 years in the West Berkshire Health Authority area during 1972–85.[15] They calculated that 45·6 cases would be expected in the area at the age specific leukaemia registration rates by calendar year for this period in England and Wales (the standard population). Using $O = 64$ and $E = 45·6$ the standardised incidence ratio (SIR) is $64/45·6 = 1·40$. Values of $O_L = 49·3$ and $O_U = 81·7$ are found from the appropriate table based on the Poisson distribution when $O = 64$ and $\alpha = 0·05$ (see Table 18.3).

The 95% confidence interval for the population value of the standardised incidence ratio is

$$\frac{49·3}{45·6} \quad \text{to} \quad \frac{81·7}{45·6}$$

that is, from 1·08 to 1·79. The uncertainty in the incidence rate in West Berkshire ranges from just 8% greater incidence to almost 80% greater incidence compared to the standard England and Wales population.

Sometimes the standardised incidence ratio (or standardised mortality ratio) is multiplied by 100 and then the same must be done to the figures describing the confidence interval.

Ratio of two standardised ratios

Let O_1 and O_2 be the observed numbers of cases (deaths) in two study groups and E_1 and E_2 the two expected numbers. It is sometimes appropriate to calculate the ratio of the two standardised incidence ratios (standardised mortality ratios) O_1/E_1 and O_2/E_2 and find a confidence interval for this ratio. Although there are known limitations to this procedure if the age-specific incidence ratios within each group to the standard are not similar, these are not serious in usual applications.[14] Again O_1 and O_2 can be regarded as Poisson variables and a confidence interval for the ratio O_1/O_2 is obtained as described by Ederer and Mantel.[16] The procedure recognises that conditional on the total of $O_1 + O_2$ the number O_1 can be considered as a Binomial variable with sample size $O_1 + O_2$ and proportion $O_1/(O_1 + O_2)$. The $100(1 - \alpha)\%$ confidence interval for the population value of the Binomial proportion can be obtained from tables based on the Binomial distribution (for example, Lentner[11]). Denote this confidence interval by A_L to A_U. The $100(1 - \alpha)\%$ confidence interval for the population value of O_1/O_2 can now be found as

$$B_L = \frac{A_L}{1 - A_L} \quad \text{to} \quad B_U = \frac{A_U}{1 - A_U}.$$

The $100(1 - \alpha)\%$ confidence interval for the population value of the ratio of the two standardised incidence ratios (standardised mortality ratios) is then given by

$$B_L \times \frac{E_2}{E_1} \quad \text{to} \quad B_U \times \frac{E_2}{E_1}.$$

Worked example

Roman *et al.* published figures for childhood leukaemia during 1972–85 in Basingstoke and North Hampshire Health Authority which gave $O = 25$ and $E = 23.7$ and a standardised incidence ratio of 1.05.[15] To compare the figures for West Berkshire from the previous example with those from Basingstoke and North Hampshire let $O_1 = 64$, $E_1 = 45.6$, $O_2 = 25$, and $E_2 = 23.7$.

The ratio of the two standardised incidence ratios is given by $(64/45.6)/(25/23.7) = 1.40/1.05 = 1.33$. From the appropriate table for the Binomial distribution with sample size of $n = 64 + 25 = 89$, proportion

$p = 64/(64 + 25) = 0.72$, and $\alpha = 0.05$, the 95% confidence interval for the population value of the Binomial proportion is found to be $A_L = 0.6138$ to $A_U = 0.8093$. The 95% confidence interval for O_1/O_2 is thus

$$\frac{0.6138}{1 - 0.6318} \quad \text{to} \quad \frac{0.8093}{1 - 0.8093}$$

that is, from 1·59 to 4·24.

The 95% confidence interval for the population value of the ratio of the two standardised incidence ratios is then given by

$$1.59 \times \frac{23.7}{45.6} \quad \text{to} \quad 4.24 \times \frac{23.7}{45.6}$$

that is, from 0·83 to 2·21.

Standardised rates

If a rate rather than a ratio is required the standardised rate (SR) in a study group is given by

$$SR = \sum N_i r_i \Big/ \sum N_i,$$

where N_i is the number of individuals in age group i of the reference population, r_i is the disease rate in age group i of the study group, and $\sum$ indicates summation over all age groups. This is usually known as the direct method of standardisation because the specific rates of the population being studied are used directly. If n_i is the number of individuals in age group i of the study group the standard error of SR can be estimated as

$$SE(SR) = \sqrt{\sum [N_i^2 r_i (1 - r_i)/n_i]} \Big/ \sum N_i.$$

This can be approximated by

$$SE(SR) = \sqrt{\sum (N_i^2 r_i/n_i)} \Big/ \sum N_i,$$

assuming that the rates r_i are small.[6]

The $100(1 - \alpha)$% confidence interval for the population value of SR is then given by

$$SR - [z_{1-\alpha/2} \times SE(SR)] \quad \text{to} \quad SR + [z_{1-\alpha/2} \times SE(SR)],$$

where $z_{1-\alpha/2}$ is the appropriate value from the Normal distribution for the $100(1 - \alpha/2)$ percentile (see Table 18.1).

Note that if the rates r_i are given as rates per 10^m (for example, $m = 3$ gives a rate per 1000), rather than as proportions, then the standardised rate (SR) is also a rate per 10^m and SE(SR) as given above needs to be multiplied by $\sqrt{10^m}$.

Worked example

The observations presented in Table 7.8 were made in a study of the radiological prevalence of Paget's disease of bone in British male migrants to Australia.[17] The standardised prevalence rate (SR) is 5·7 per 100 with SE$(SR) = 1·17$ per 100.

Table 7.8 Paget's disease of bone in British male migrants to Australia by age group[17]

| Age (years) | Study group | | | Standard population (N_i)[18] |
	Cases	n_i	Rate per 100 (r_i)	
55–64	4	96	4·2	2773
65–74	13	237	5·5	2556
75–84	8	105	7·6	1113
≥85	7	32	21·9	184
Totals	32	470	6·8	6626

The 95% confidence interval for the population value of the standardised prevalence rate is then given by

$$5·7 - (1·96 \times 1·17) \quad \text{to} \quad 5·7 + (1·96 \times 1·17)$$

that is, from 3·5 to 8·0 per 100.

Comment

Many of the methods described here and others are also given with examples by Rothman and Greenland.[19] Several alternative methods of constructing confidence intervals for standardised rates and ratios have been developed.[20–23] Further discussion of confidence limits for the relative risk can be found in Bailey.[24] In particular, a method based on likelihood scores is evaluated by Gart and Nam[25] (see also chapter 10). A useful review of approximate confidence intervals for relative risks and odds ratios is given by Sato.[26]

1 Katz D, Baptista J, Azen SP, Pike MC. Obtaining confidence intervals for the risk ratio in cohort studies. *Biometrics* 1978;**34**:469–74.
2 Brenner H, Rothenbacher D, Bode G, Adler G. Parental history of gastric or duodenal ulcer and prevalence of *Helicobacter pylori* infection in preschool children: population based study. *BMJ* 1998;**316**:665.

3 Daly LE. Confidence limits made easy: interval estimation using a substitution method. *Am J Epidemiol* 1998;**147**:783–90.

4 Greenland S. Re: "Confidence limits made easy: Interval estimation using a substitution method". *Am J Epidemiol* 1999;**149**:884.

5 Walter SD. The estimation and interpretation of attributable risk in health research. *Biometrics* 1976;**32**:829–49.

6 Armitage P, Berry G. *Statistical methods in medical research.* 3rd edn. Oxford: Blackwell, 1994: 438, 509, 512, 514.

7 Woolf B. On estimating the relationship between blood group and disease. *Ann Hum Genet* 1955;**19**:251–3.

8 Breslow NE, Day NE. *Statistical methods in cancer research. Volume 1—The analysis of case-control studies.* Lyon: International Agency for Research on Cancer, 1980: 124–146, 169–182, 192–246.

9 Shinebaum R, Blackwell CC, Forster PJG, Hurst NP, Weir DM, Nuki G. Non-secretion of ABO blood group antigens as a host susceptibility factor in the spondyloarthropathies. *BMJ* 1987;**294**:208–10.

10 Wald NJ, Nanchahal K, Thompson SG, Cuckle HS. Does breathing other people's tobacco smoke cause lung cancer? *BMJ* 1986;**293**:1217–22.

11 Lentner C, ed. *Geigy scientific tables.* Volume 2. 8th edn. Basle: Ciba-Geigy, 1982:89–102.

12 Eason J, Markowe HLJ. Controlled investigation of deaths from asthma in hospitals in the North East Thames region. *BMJ* 1987;**294**:1255–8.

13 Nunn AJ, Mulder DW, Kamali A, Ruberantwari A, Kengeya-Kayondo J-F, Whitworth J. Mortality associated with HIV-1 infection over five years in a rural Ugandan population: cohort study. *BMJ* 1997;**315**:767–71.

14 Breslow NE, Day NE. *Statistical methods in cancer research. Volume 2—The design and analysis of cohort studies.* Oxford: Oxford University Press, 1988: 69, 93.

15 Roman E, Beral V, Carpenter L, *et al.* Childhood leukaemia in the West Berkshire and the Basingstoke and North Hampshire District Health Authorities in relation to nuclear establishments in the vicinity. *BMJ* 1987;**294**:597–602.

16 Ederer F, Mantel N. Confidence limits on the ratio of two Poisson variables. *Am J Epidemiol* 1974;**100**:165–7.

17 Gardner MJ, Guyer PB, Barker DJP. Radiological prevalence of Paget's disease of bone in British migrants to Australia. *BMJ* 1978;**i**:1655–7.

18 Barker DJP, Clough PWL, Guyer PB, Gardner MJ. Paget's disease of bone in 14 British towns. *BMJ* 1977;**i**:1181–3.

19 Rothman KJ, Greenland S. *Modern epidemiology.* 2nd edn. Philadelphia: Lippincott-Raven, 1998; chapters 14–16.

20 Ulm K. A simple method to calculate the confidence interval of a standardized mortality ratio (SMR). *Am J Epidemiol* 1990;**131**:373–5.

21 Sahai H, Khurshid A. Confidence intervals for the mean of a Poisson distribution: a review. *Biom J* 1993;7:857–67.

22 Fay MP, Feuer EJ. Confidence intervals for directly standardized rates: a method based on the gamma distribution. *Statist Med* 1997;**16**:791–801.

23 Kulkarni PM, Tripathi RC, Michalek JE. Maximum (max) and mid-p confidence intervals and p values for the standardized mortality and incidence ratios. *Am J Epidemiol* 1998;**147**:83–6.

24 Bailey BJR. Confidence limits to the risk ratio. *Biometrics* 1987;**43**:201–5.

25 Gart JJ, Nam J. Approximate interval estimation of the ratio of binomial parameters: A review and corrections for skewness. *Biometrics* 1988;**44**:323–38.

26 Sato T. Confidence intervals for effect parameters common in cancer epidemiology. *Environ Health Perspect* 1990;**87**:95–101.

8 Regression and correlation

DOUGLAS G ALTMAN, MARTIN J GARDNER

The most common statistical analyses are those that examine one or two groups of individuals with respect to a single variable (see chapters 4 to 7). Also common are those analyses that consider the relation between two variables in one group of subjects. We use regression analysis to predict one variable from another, and correlation analysis to see if the values of two variables are associated. The purposes of these two analyses are distinct, and usually one only should be used.

We outline the calculation of the linear regression equation for predicting one variable from another and show how to calculate confidence intervals for the population value of the slope and intercept of the line, for the line itself, and for predictions made using the regression equation. We explain how to obtain a confidence interval for the population value of the difference between the slopes of regression lines from two groups of subjects and how to calculate a confidence interval for the vertical distance between two parallel regression lines.

We also describe the calculations of confidence intervals for Pearson's correlation coefficient and Spearman's rank correlation coefficient.

The calculations have been carried out to full arithmetical precision, as is recommended practice (see chapter 14), but intermediate steps are shown as rounded results. Methods of calculating confidence intervals for different aspects of regression and correlation are demonstrated. The appropriate ones to use depend on the particular problem being studied.

The interpretation of confidence intervals has been discussed in chapters 1 and 3. Confidence intervals convey only the effects of sampling variation on the estimated statistics and cannot control for other errors such as biases in design, conduct, or analysis.

Linear regression analysis

For two variables x and y we wish to calculate the regression equation for predicting y from x. We call y the dependent or outcome variable and x the independent or explanatory variable. The equation for the population regression line is

$$y = A + Bx$$

where A is the intercept on the vertical y axis (the value of y when $x = 0$) and B is the slope of the line. In standard regression analysis it is assumed that the distribution of the y variable at each value of x is Normal with the same standard deviation, but no assumptions are made about the distribution of the x variable. Sample estimates a (of A) and b (of B) are needed and also the means of the two variables ($\bar{x}$ and $\bar{y}$), the standard deviations of the two variables (s_x and s_y), and the residual standard deviation of y about the regression line (s_{res}). The formulae for deriving a, b, and s_{res} are given under "Technical details" at the end of this chapter.

All the following confidence intervals associated with a single regression line use the quantity $t_{1-\alpha/2}$, the appropriate value from the t distribution with $n - 2$ degrees of freedom where n is the sample size. Thus, for a 95% confidence interval we need the value that cuts off the top 2·5% of the t distribution, denoted $t_{0.975}$.

A fitted regression line should be used to make predictions only within the observed range of the x variable. Extrapolation outside this range is unwarranted and may mislead.[1]

It is always advisable to plot the data to see whether a linear relationship between x and y is reasonable. In addition a plot of the "residuals" ("observed minus predicted"—see "Technical details" at the end of this chapter) is useful to check the distributional assumptions for the y variable.

Illustrative data set

Table 8.1 shows data from a clinical trial of enalapril versus placebo in diabetic patients.[2] The variables studied are mean arterial blood pressure (mmHg) and total glycosylated haemoglobin concentration (%). The analyses presented here are illustrative and do not relate directly to the clinical trial. Most of the methods

74

Table 8.1 Mean arterial blood pressure and total glycosylated haemoglobin concentration in two groups of 10 diabetics on entry to a clinical trial of enalapril versus placebo[2]

Enalapril group		Placebo group	
Mean arterial blood pressure (mmHg) x	Total glycosylated haemoglobin (%) y	Mean arterial blood pressure (mmHg) x	Total glycosylated haemoglobin (%) y
91	9·8	98	9·5
104	7·4	105	6·7
107	7·9	100	7·0
107	8·3	101	8·6
106	8·3	99	6·7
100	9·0	87	9·5
92	9·7	98	9·0
92	8·8	104	7·6
105	7·6	106	8·5
108	6·9	90	8·6
Means:			
$\bar{x} = 101\cdot2$	$\bar{y} = 8\cdot37$	$\bar{x} = 98\cdot8$	$\bar{y} = 8\cdot17$
Standard deviations:			
$s_x = 6\cdot941$	$s_y = 0\cdot9615$	$s_x = 6\cdot161$	$s_y = 1\cdot0914$
Standard deviations about the fitted regression lines:			
	$s_{res} = 0\cdot5485$		$s_{res} = 0\cdot9866$

for calculating confidence intervals are demonstrated using only the data from the 10 subjects who received enalapril.

Single sample

We want to describe the way total glycosylated haemoglobin concentration changes with mean arterial blood pressure. The regression line of total glycosylated haemoglobin (TGH) concentration on mean arterial blood pressure (MAP) for the 10 subjects receiving enalapril is found to be

$$TGH = 20\cdot19 - 0\cdot1168 \times MAP.$$

The estimated slope of the line is negative, indicating lower total glycosylated haemoglobin concentrations for subjects with higher mean arterial blood pressure.

The other quantities needed to obtain the various confidence intervals are shown in Table 8.1. The calculations use 95% confidence intervals. For this we need the value of $t_{0.975}$ with 8 degrees of freedom, and Table 18.2 shows this to be 2·306.

Confidence interval for the slope of the regression line

The slope of the sample regression line estimates the mean change in y for a unit change in x. The standard error of the slope, b, is calculated as

$$\text{SE}(b) = \frac{s_{\text{res}}}{s_x \sqrt{n-1}}.$$

The $100(1 - \alpha)\%$ confidence interval for the population value of the slope, B, is given by

$$b - [t_{1-\alpha/2} \times \text{SE}(b)] \quad \text{to} \quad b + [t_{1-\alpha/2} \times \text{SE}(b)].$$

Worked example

The standard error of the slope is

$$\text{SE}(b) = \frac{0.5845}{6.941 \times \sqrt{9}} = 0.02634\% \text{ per mmHg}.$$

The 95% confidence interval for the population value of the slope is thus

$$-0.1168 - (2.306 \times 0.02634) \quad \text{to} \quad -0.1168 + (2.306 \times 0.02634)$$

that is, from -0.178 to -0.056% per mmHg.

For brevity, in further calculations on these data we will describe the units as %.

Confidence interval for the mean value of y for a given value of x and for the regression line

The estimated mean value of y for any chosen value of x, say x_0, is obtained from the fitted regression line as

$$y_{\text{fit}} = a + bx_0.$$

The standard error of y_{fit} is given by

$$\text{SE}(y_{\text{fit}}) = s_{\text{res}} \times \sqrt{\frac{1}{n} + \frac{(x_0 - \bar{x})^2}{(n-1)s_x^2}}.$$

The $100(1 - \alpha)\%$ confidence interval for the population mean value of y at $x = x_0$ is then

$$y_{\text{fit}} - [t_{1-\alpha/2} \times \text{SE}(y_{\text{fit}})] \quad \text{to} \quad y_{\text{fit}} + [t_{1-\alpha/2} \times \text{SE}(y_{\text{fit}})].$$

When this calculation is made for all values of x in the observed range of x a $100(1 - \alpha)\%$ confidence interval for the position of the population regression line is obtained. Because of the expression $(x_0 - \bar{x})^2$ in the formula for $\text{SE}(y_{\text{fit}})$ the confidence interval becomes wider with increasing distance of x_0 from $\bar{x}$.

The confidence interval for the mean total glycosylated haemoglobin concentration can be calculated for any specified value of mean arterial blood pressure. If the mean arterial blood pressure of interest is 100 mmHg the estimated total glycosylated haemoglobin concentration is $y_{fit} = 20\cdot19 - (0\cdot1168 \times 100) = 8\cdot51\%$. The standard error of this estimated value is

$$\mathrm{SE}(y_{fit}) = 0\cdot5485 \times \sqrt{\frac{1}{10} + \frac{(100 - 101\cdot2)^2}{9 \times 6\cdot941^2}} = 0\cdot1763\%.$$

The 95% confidence interval for the mean total glycosylated haemoglobin concentration for the population of diabetic subjects with a mean arterial blood pressure of 100 mmHg is thus

$$8\cdot51 - (2\cdot306 \times 0\cdot1763) \quad \text{to} \quad 8\cdot51 + (2\cdot306 \times 0\cdot1763),$$

that is, from 8·10% to 8·92%.

By calculating the 95% confidence interval for the mean total glycosylated haemoglobin concentration for all values of mean arterial blood pressure within the range of observations we get a 95% confidence interval for the population regression line. This is shown in Figure 8.1.

The confidence interval becomes wider as the mean arterial blood pressure moves away from the mean of 101·2 mmHg.

Confidence interval for the intercept of the regression line

The intercept of the regression line on the y axis is generally of less interest than the slope of the line and does not usually have any obvious clinical interpretation. It can be seen that the intercept is the fitted value of y when x is zero.

Thus a $100(1 - \alpha)\%$ confidence interval for the population value of the intercept, A, can be obtained using the formula from the preceding section with $x_0 = 0$ and $y_{fit} = a$. The standard error of a is given by

$$\mathrm{SE}(a) = s_{res} \times \sqrt{\frac{1}{n} + \frac{(\bar{x})^2}{(n - 1)s_x^2}}.$$

The confidence interval for a is thus given by

$$a - [t_{1 - \alpha/2} \times \mathrm{SE}(a)] \quad \text{to} \quad a + [t_{1 - \alpha/2} \times \mathrm{SE}(a)].$$

The confidence interval for the population value of the intercept is the confidence interval for y_{fit} when $x = 0$, and is calculated as before. In this

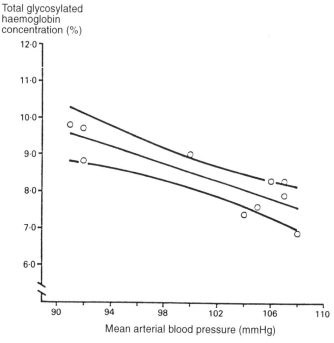

Figure 8.1 Regression line of total glycosylated haemoglobin concentration on mean arterial blood pressure, with 95% confidence interval for the population mean total glycosylated haemoglobin concentration.

case the intercept is 20·19%, with a standard error of 2·67%. Thus the 95% confidence interval is from 14·03% to 26·35%. Clearly in this example the intercept, relating to a mean arterial blood pressure of zero, is extrapolated well below the range of the data and is of no interest in itself.

Prediction interval for an individual (and all individuals)

It is useful to calculate the uncertainty in y_{fit} as a predictor of y for an individual. The range of uncertainty is called a prediction (or tolerance) interval. A prediction interval is wider than the associated confidence interval for the mean value of y because the scatter of data about the regression line is more important. Unlike the confidence interval for the slope, the width of the prediction interval is not greatly influenced by sample size.

For an individual whose value of x is x_0 the predicted value of y is y_{fit}, given by

$$y_{fit} = a + bx_0.$$

To calculate the prediction interval we first estimate the standard deviation (s_{pred}) of individual values of y when x equals x_0 as

$$s_{pred} = s_{res} \times \sqrt{1 + \frac{1}{n} + \frac{(x_0 - \bar{x})^2}{(n-1)s_x^2}}.$$

The $100(1 - \alpha)\%$ prediction interval is then

$$y_{fit} - (t_{1-\alpha/2} \times s_{pred}) \quad \text{to} \quad y_{fit} + (t_{1-\alpha/2} \times s_{pred}).$$

When this calculation is made for all values of x in the observed range the estimated prediction interval should include the values of y for $100(1 - \alpha)\%$ of subjects in the population.

Worked example

The 95% prediction interval for the total glycosylated haemoglobin concentration of an individual subject with a mean arterial blood pressure of 100 mmHg is obtained by first calculating s_{pred}:

$$s_{pred} = 0{\cdot}5485 \times \sqrt{1 + \frac{1}{10} + \frac{(100 - 101{\cdot}2)^2}{9 \times 6{\cdot}941^2}} = 0{\cdot}5761\%.$$

The 95% prediction interval is then given by

$$8{\cdot}51 - (2{\cdot}306 \times 0{\cdot}5761) \quad \text{to} \quad 8{\cdot}51 + (2{\cdot}306 \times 0{\cdot}5761)$$

that is, from 7·18 to 9·84%.

The contrast with the narrower 95% confidence interval for the mean total glycosylated haemoglobin concentration for a mean arterial blood pressure of 100 mmHg calculated above is noticeable. The 95% prediction intervals for the range of observed levels of mean arterial blood pressure are shown in Figure 8.2 and again these widen on moving away from the mean arterial blood pressure of 101·2 mmHg.

Two samples

Regression lines fitted to observations from two independent groups of subjects can be analysed to see if they come from populations with regression lines that are parallel or even coincident.[3]

Confidence interval for the difference between the slopes of two regression lines

If we have fitted regression lines to two different sets of data on the same two variables we can construct a confidence interval for the difference between the population regression slopes using a similar approach to that for a single regression line. The standard

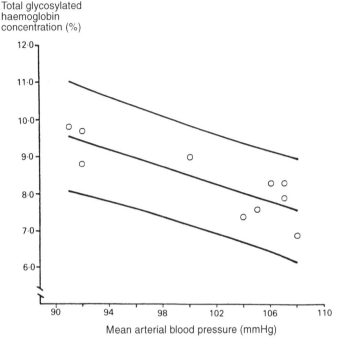

Figure 8.2 Regression line of total glycosylated haemoglobin concentration on mean arterial blood pressure, with 95% prediction interval for an individual total glycosylated haemoglobin concentration.

error of the difference between the slopes is given by first calculating s_{pool}, the pooled residual standard deviation, as

$$s_{\text{pool}} = \sqrt{\frac{(n_1 - 2)s_{\text{res}_1}^2 + (n_2 - 2)s_{\text{res}_2}^2}{n_1 + n_2 - 4}}$$

and then

$$\text{SE}(b_1 - b_2) = s_{\text{pool}} \times \sqrt{\frac{1}{(n_1 - 1)s_{x_1}^2} + \frac{1}{(n_2 - 1)s_{x_2}^2}},$$

where the suffixes 1 and 2 indicate values derived from the two separate sets of data. The $100(1 - \alpha)\%$ confidence interval for the population difference between the slopes is now given by

$$b_1 - b_2 - [t_{1-\alpha/2} \times \text{SE}(b_1 - b_2)] \quad \text{to}$$

$$b_1 - b_2 + [t_{1-\alpha/2} \times \text{SE}(b_1 - b_2)]$$

where $t_{1-\alpha/2}$ is the appropriate value from the t distribution with $n_1 + n_2 - 4$ degrees of freedom.

Worked example

The regression line for the placebo group from the data in Table 8.1 is

$$\text{TGH} = 17{\cdot}33 - 0{\cdot}09268 \times \text{MAP}.$$

The difference between the estimated slopes of the two regression lines is $-0{\cdot}1168 - (-0{\cdot}09268) = -0{\cdot}02412\%$. The standard error of this difference is found by first calculating s_{pool} as

$$s_{\text{pool}} = \sqrt{\frac{8 \times 0{\cdot}5485^2 + 8 \times 0{\cdot}9866^2}{16}} = 0{\cdot}7982\%,$$

and then

$$\text{SE}(b_1 - b_2) = 0{\cdot}7982 \times \sqrt{\frac{1}{9 \times 6{\cdot}941^2} + \frac{1}{9 \times 6{\cdot}161^2}} = 0{\cdot}05774\%.$$

From Table 18.2 the value of $t_{0.975}$ with 16 degrees of freedom is $2{\cdot}120$, so the 95% confidence interval for the population difference between the slopes is

$$-0{\cdot}02412 - (2{\cdot}120 \times 0{\cdot}05774) \quad \text{to} \quad -0{\cdot}02412 + (2{\cdot}120 \times 0{\cdot}05774)$$

that is, from $-0{\cdot}147$ to $0{\cdot}098\%$.

Since a zero difference between slopes is near the middle of this confidence interval there is no evidence that the two population regression lines have different slopes. This is not surprising in this example as the subjects were allocated at random to the treatment groups.

Confidence interval for the common slope of two parallel regression lines

If the chosen confidence interval—for example, 95%—for the difference between population values of the slopes includes zero it is reasonable to fit two parallel regression lines with the same slope and calculate a confidence interval for their common slope. In practice we would usually perform this analysis by multiple regression using a statistical software package (see below). The calculation can be done, however, using the results obtained by fitting separate regression lines to the two groups and the standard deviations of the x and y values in the two groups: s_{x_1}, s_{x_2}, s_{y_1}, and s_{y_2}. First we define the quantity w as

$$w = (n_1 - 1)s_{x_1}^2 + (n_2 - 1)s_{x_2}^2.$$

The common slope of the parallel lines (b_{par}) is estimated as

$$b_{\text{par}} = \frac{b_1(n_1 - 1)s_{x_1}^2 + b_2(n_2 - 1)s_{x_2}^2}{w}.$$

The residual standard deviation of y around the parallel lines (s_{par}) is given by

$$s_{par} = \sqrt{\frac{(n_1 - 1)s_{y_1}^2 + (n_2 - 1)s_{y_2}^2 - b_{par}^2 \times w}{n_1 + n_2 - 3}}$$

and the standard error of the slope by

$$SE(b_{par}) = \frac{s_{par}}{\sqrt{w}}.$$

The $100(1 - \alpha)\%$ confidence interval for the population value of the common slope is then

$$b_{par} - [t_{1 - \alpha/2} \times SE(b_{par})] \quad \text{to} \quad b_{par} + [t_{1 - \alpha/2} \times SE(b_{par})],$$

where $t_{1 - \alpha/2}$ is the appropriate value from the t distribution with $n_1 + n_2 - 3$ degrees of freedom.

Worked example

We first calculate the quantity w as

$$w = 9 \times 6 \cdot 941^2 + 9 \times 6 \cdot 161^2 = 775 \cdot 22.$$

The common slope of the parallel lines is then found as

$$b_{par} = \frac{-0 \cdot 1168 \times 9 \times 6 \cdot 941^2 + (-0 \cdot 09268) \times 9 \times 6 \cdot 161^2}{775 \cdot 22}$$

$$= -0 \cdot 1062\%.$$

The residual standard deviation of y around the parallel lines is

$$s_{par} = \sqrt{\frac{9 \times 0 \cdot 9615^2 + 9 \times 1 \cdot 0914^2 - (-0 \cdot 1062)^2 \times 775 \cdot 22}{10 + 10 - 3}}$$

$$= 0 \cdot 7786\%.$$

The standard error of the common slope is thus

$$SE(b_{par}) = \frac{0 \cdot 7786}{\sqrt{775 \cdot 22}} = 0 \cdot 02796\%.$$

From Table 18.2 the value of $t_{1 - \alpha/2}$ with 17 degrees of freedom is $2 \cdot 110$, so that the 95% confidence interval for the population value of b_{par} is therefore

$$0 \cdot 1062 - (2 \cdot 110 \times 0 \cdot 02796) \quad \text{to} \quad -0 \cdot 1062 + (2 \cdot 110 \times 0 \cdot 02796)$$

that is, from $-0 \cdot 165$ to $-0 \cdot 047\%$.

Confidence interval for the vertical distance between two parallel regression lines

The intercepts of the two parallel lines with the y axis are given by

$$\bar{y}_1 - b_{\text{par}}\bar{x}_1 \quad \text{and} \quad \bar{y}_2 - b_{\text{par}}\bar{x}_2.$$

We are usually more interested in the difference between the intercepts, which is the vertical distance between the parallel lines. This is the same as the difference between the fitted y values for the two groups at the same value of x, and is equivalent to adjusting the observed mean values of y for the mean values of x, a method known as analysis of covariance.[3] The adjusted mean difference (y_{diff}) is calculated as

$$y_{\text{diff}} = \bar{y}_1 - \bar{y}_2 - b_{\text{par}}(\bar{x}_1 - \bar{x}_2)$$

and the standard error of y_{diff} is

$$\text{SE}(y_{\text{diff}}) = s_{\text{par}} \times \sqrt{\frac{1}{n_1} + \frac{1}{n_2} + \frac{(\bar{x}_1 - \bar{x}_2)^2}{w}}.$$

The $100(1 - \alpha)\%$ confidence interval for the population value of y_{diff} is then

$$y_{\text{diff}} - [t_{1-\alpha/2} \times \text{SE}(y_{\text{diff}})] \quad \text{to} \quad y_{\text{diff}} + [t_{1-\alpha/2} \times \text{SE}(y_{\text{diff}})]$$

where $t_{1-\alpha/2}$ is the appropriate value from the t distribution with $n_1 + n_2 - 3$ degrees of freedom.

Worked example

Using the calculated value for the common slope the adjusted difference between the mean total glycosylated haemoglobin concentration in the two groups is

$$y_{\text{diff}} = (8.37 - 8.17) - (-0.1062) \times (101.2 - 98.8) = 0.4548\%,$$

and its standard error is

$$\text{SE}(y_{\text{diff}}) = 0.7786 \times \sqrt{\frac{1}{10} + \frac{1}{10} + \frac{(101.2 - 98.8)^2}{775.22}} = 0.3546\%.$$

The 95% confidence interval for the population value of y_{diff} is then given by

$$0.4548 - (2.110 \times 0.3546) \quad \text{to} \quad 0.4548 + (2.110 \times 0.3546)$$

that is, from -0.29 to 1.20%.

Figure 8·3 illustrates the effect of adjustment.

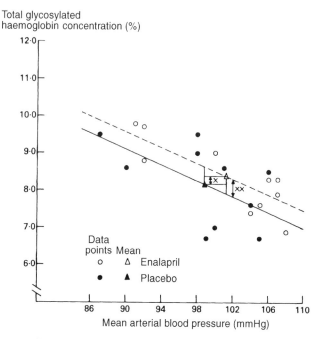

Figure 8.3 Ilustration of the calculation of the adjusted difference between mean total glycosylated haemoglobin concentrations in two groups.
Differences between means:
$\times$, observed difference $= \bar{y}_1 - \bar{y}_2 = 0.20\%$;
$\times\times$, adjusted difference $= y_{\text{diff}} = 0.45\%$.

More than two samples

The methods described for two groups can be extended to the case of more than two groups of individuals,[3] although such problems are rather rare. The calculations are best done using software for multiple regression, as discussed below.

We have shown linear regression with a continuous explanatory variable but this is not a requirement. Regression with a single binary explanatory variable is equivalent to performing a two-sample t test. When several explanatory variables are considered at once using multiple regression, as described below, it is common for some to be binary.

Binary outcome variable—logistic regression

In many studies the outcome variable of interest is the presence or absence of some condition, such as responding to treatment or having a myocardial infarction. When we have a binary outcome variable and give the categories numerical values of 0 and 1, usually representing "No" and "Yes" respectively, then the mean of these values in a sample of individuals is the same as the proportion of individuals with the characteristic. We might expect, therefore, that the appropriate regression model would predict the proportion of subjects with the feature of interest (or, equivalently, the probability of an individual having that characteristic) for different values of the explanatory variable.

The basic principle of logistic regression is much the same as for ordinary multiple regression. The main difference is that the model predicts a transformation of the outcome of interest. If p is the proportion of individuals with the characteristic, the transformation we use is the logit transformation, $\mathrm{logit}(p) = \log[p/(1-p)]$. The regression coefficient for an explanatory variable compares the estimated outcome associated with two values of that variable, and is the log of the odds ratio (see chapter 7). We can thus use the model to estimate the odds ratio as e^b, where b is the estimated regression coefficient (log odds ratio). A confidence interval for the odds ratio is obtained by applying the same transformation to the confidence interval for the regression coefficient. An example is given below, in the section on multiple regression.

Outcome is time to an event—Cox regression

The regression method introduced by Cox in 1972 is used widely when the outcome is the time to an event.[4] It is also known as proportional hazards regression analysis. The underlying methodology is complex, but the resulting regression model has a similar interpretation to a logistic regression model. Again the explanatory variable could be continuous or binary (for example, treatment in a randomised trial).

In this model the regression coefficient is the logarithm of the relative hazard (or "hazard ratio") at a given time. The hazard represents the risk of the event in a very short time interval after a given time, given survival that far. The hazard ratio is interpreted as the relative risk of the event for two groups defined by different values of the explanatory variable. The model makes the strong assumption that this ratio is the same at all times after the start of follow up (for example, after randomisation in a controlled trial).

We can use the model to estimate the hazard ratio as e^b, where b is the estimated regression coefficient (log hazard ratio). As for logistic regression, a confidence interval is obtained by applying the same transformation to the confidence interval for the regression coefficient. An example is given below, in the section on multiple regression. A more detailed explanation of the method is given in chapter 9.

Several explanatory variables—multiple regression

In much medical research there are several potential explanatory variables. The principles of regression—linear, logistic, or Cox—can be extended fairly simply by using multiple regression.[4] Further, the analysis may include binary as well as continuous explanatory variables. Standard statistical software can perform such calculations in a straightforward way. There are many issues relating to such analysis that are beyond the scope of this book—for discussion see, for example, Altman.[4]

Although the nature of the prediction varies according to the model, in each case the multiple regression analysis produces a regression equation (or "model") which is effectively a weighted combination of the explanatory variables. The regression coefficients are the weights given to each variable.

For each variable in the regression model there is a standard error, so that it is easy to calculate a confidence interval for any particular variable in the model, using the standard approach of chapter 3.

The multiple linear regression model is

$$Y = b_0 + b_1 X_1 + b_2 X_2 + \ldots + b_k X_k,$$

where Y is the outcome variable, X_1 to X_k are k explanatory variables, b_0 is a constant (intercept), and b_1 to b_k are the regression coefficients. The nature of the predicted outcome, Y, varies according to the type of model, as discussed above, but the regression model has the same form in each case. The main difference in multiple regression is that the relation between the outcome and a particular explanatory variable is "adjusted" for the effects of other variables.

The explanatory variables can be either continuous or binary. Table 8.2 shows the interpretation of regression coefficients for different types of outcome variable and for either continuous or

Table 8.2 Interpretation of regression coefficients for different types of outcome variable and for either continuous or binary explanatory variables

Type of outcome variable (Y)	Type of multiple regression	Continuous explanatory variable (X)	Binary explanatory variable (X)
Continuous	Linear	Change in Y for a unit change in X	Difference between mean of Y in two groups
Binary	Logistic	Log odds ratio associated with a unit change in X	Log odds ratio
Time to event	Cox (proportional hazards)	Log hazard ratio associated with a unit change in X	Log hazard ratio

binary explanatory variables. For binary variables it is assumed that these have numerical codes that differ by one; most often these are 0 and 1.

For multiple logistic regression models the regression coefficients and their confidence intervals need to be exponentiated (antilogged) to give the estimated odds ratio and its confidence interval. The same process is needed in Cox regression to get the estimated hazard ratio with its confidence interval.

Examples

Table 8.3 shows a multiple logistic regression model from a study of 183 men with unstable angina.[5] The regression coefficients and confidence intervals have been converted to the odds ratio scale.

Some points to note about this analysis are:

- The odds ratio for a binary variable (all here except age) indicates the estimated increased risk of the outcome for those with the feature. (The interpretation of an odds ratio as an approximate relative risk depends on the event being reasonably rare.)

Table 8.3 Logistic regression model for predicting cardiac death or non-fatal myocardial infarction.[5]

Variable	Odds ratio	95% CI
Diabetes mellitus	4·56	1·51 to 13·7
Age	1·08	1·02 to 1·14
Previous myocardial infarction	2·83	1·06 to 7·57
Troponin T status	1·21	0·42 to 3·47
Further pain or electrographic changes, or both	0·84	0·31 to 2·29

Table 8.4 Association between number of children and risk of testicular cancer in Danish men (514 cases and 720 controls)[6]

No. of children	Adjusted odds ratio (95% CI)
0	1·00
1	0·75 (0·51 to 1·10)
2	0·68 (0·47 to 0·98)
≥3	0·52 (0·32 to 0·85)

- For two of the binary variables, diabetes and previous myocardial infarction, the confidence interval excludes 1, suggesting that these are indeed risk factors.
- The odds ratio for age represents the increased risk per extra year of age. Thus, for example, the model predicts that a 70-year-old man has about an 8% extra risk of a serious cardiac event compared to a 69-year-old man. For a ten-year age difference the estimated odds ratio is $1·08^{10}$ or 2·16, representing over a twofold risk or a 116% higher risk. The confidence interval for a ten-year difference is from $1·02^{10}$ to $1·22^{10}$, that is 1·22 to 7·30.
- The variables were included in this model if they showed a significant association with the outcome in a univariate (unadjusted) analysis. Although common, this procedure may lead to biased estimates of effect and the confidence intervals will be too narrow. The same comment applies to the use of stepwise selection within the multiple regression. (These remarks apply to all types of multiple regression.)
- The data are actually times to a specific event and could (and perhaps should) have been analysed using Cox regression (chapter 9).

Table 8.4 shows part of a multiple logistic regression model with an ordinal explanatory variable. The number of children was compared for men with testicular cancer and controls, and adjustment made in the model for cryptorchidism, testicular atrophy, and other characteristics. Here each group with children is compared with the reference group with no children. This is achieved in the regression model by creating three binary variables indicating respectively whether or not each man has 1, 2, or 3 children. At most one of these 'dummy' variables will be 1, and the others are zero.[4]

Note that the overall evaluation of the relation between this ordinal variable and outcome (here risk of testicular cancer) should be based on the trend across the four groups (see "Multiple comparisons" in chapter 13). Here there was a highly significant trend of decreasing risk in relation to number of children even though one of the confidence intervals does not exclude 1.[6]

Correlation analysis

Pearson's product moment correlation coefficient

The correlation coefficient usually calculated is the product moment correlation coefficient or Pearson's r. This measures the degree of linear 'co-relation' between two variables x and y. The formula for calculating r for a sample of observations is given at the end of the chapter.

A confidence interval for the population value of r can be constructed by using a transformation of r to a quantity Z, which has an approximately Normal distribution. This calculation relies on the assumption that x and y have a joint bivariate Normal distribution (in practice, that the distributions of both variables are reasonably Normal).

The transformed value, Z, is given by

$$Z = \frac{1}{2} \log_e \left(\frac{1+r}{1-r} \right),$$

which for all values of r has $\text{SE} = 1/\sqrt{n-3}$ where n is the sample size. For a $100(1-\alpha)\%$ confidence interval we then calculate the two quantities

$$F = Z - \frac{z_{1-\alpha/2}}{\sqrt{n-3}} \quad \text{and} \quad G = Z + \frac{z_{1-\alpha/2}}{\sqrt{n-3}}$$

where $z_{1-\alpha/2}$ is the appropriate value from the standard Normal distribution for the $100(1-\alpha/2)$ percentile (Table 18.1).

The values F and G need to be transformed back to the original scale to give a $100(1-\alpha)\%$ confidence interval for the population correlation coefficient as

$$\frac{e^{2F}-1}{e^{2F}+1} \quad \text{to} \quad \frac{e^{2G}-1}{e^{2G}+1}.$$

Worked example

Table 8.5 shows the basal metabolic rate and total energy expenditure in 24 hours from a study of 13 non-obese women.[7] The data are ranked by increasing basal metabolic rate. Pearson's r for these data is 0·7283, and the transformed value Z is

$$Z = \frac{1}{2} \log_e \left(\frac{1+0\cdot7283}{1-0\cdot7283} \right) = 0\cdot9251.$$

89

Table 8.5 Basal metabolic rate and isotopically measured 24-hour energy expenditure in 13 non-obese women[7]

Basal metabolic rate (MJ/day)	24-hour total energy expenditure (MJ)
4·67	7·05
5·06	6·13
5·31	8·09
5·37	8·08
5·54	7·53
5·65	7·58
5·76	8·40
5·85	7·48
5·86	7·48
5·90	8·11
5·91	7·90
6·19	10·88
6·40	10·15

The values of F and G for a 95% confidence interval are

$$F = 0.9251 - \frac{1.96}{\sqrt{10}} = 0.3053$$

and

$$G = 0.9251 + \frac{1.96}{\sqrt{10}} = 1.545.$$

From these values we derive the 95% confidence interval for the population correlation coefficient as

$$\frac{e^{2 \times 0.3053} - 1}{e^{2 \times 0.3053} + 1} \quad \text{to} \quad \frac{e^{2 \times 1.545} - 1}{e^{2 \times 1.545} + 1}$$

that is, from 0·30 to 0·91.

Spearman's rank correlation coefficient

If either the distributional assumptions are not met or the relation between x and y is not linear we can use a rank method to assess a more general relation between the values of x and y. To calculate Spearman's rank correlation coefficient (r_s) the values of x and y for the n individuals have to be ranked separately in order of increasing size from 1 to n. Spearman's rank correlation coefficient is then obtained either by using the standard formula for Pearson's product moment correlation coefficient on the ranks of the two variables, or (as shown below under "Technical details") using the difference in their two ranks for each individual.

The distribution of r_s similar to that of Pearson's r, so that confidence intervals can be constructed as shown in the previous section.

Technical details: formulae for regression and correlation analyses

We strongly recommend that statistical software is used to perform regression or correlation analyses. Some formulae are given here to help explain the underlying principles.

Regression

The slope of the regression line is given by

$$b = \left(\sum xy - n\bar{x}\bar{y}\right) \Big/ \left(\sum x^2 - n\bar{x}^2\right),$$

where $\sum$ represents summation over the sample of size n. The intercept is given by

$$a = \bar{y} - b\bar{x}.$$

The difference between the observed and predicted values of y for an individual with observed values x_0 and y_0 is $y_0 - y_{\text{fit}}$, where $y_{\text{fit}} = a + bx_0$. The standard deviation of these differences (called "residuals") is thus a measure of how well the line fits the data.

The residual standard deviation of y about the regression line is

$$\begin{aligned}
s_{\text{res}} &= \sqrt{\frac{\sum(y - y_{\text{fit}})^2}{n - 2}} \\
&= \sqrt{\frac{\sum y^2 - n\bar{y}^2 - b^2(\sum x^2 - n\bar{x}^2)}{n - 2}} \\
&= \sqrt{\frac{(n - 1)(s_y^2 - b^2 s_x^2)}{n - 2}}.
\end{aligned}$$

Most statistical computer programs give all the necessary quantities to derive confidence intervals, but you may find that the output refers to s_{res} as the 'standard error of the estimate'.

Correlation

The correlation coefficient (Pearson's r) is estimated by

$$r = \left(\sum xy - n\bar{x}\bar{y}\right) \Big/ \sqrt{\left(\sum x^2 - n\bar{x}^2\right)\left(\sum y^2 - n\bar{y}^2\right)}.$$

Spearman's rank correlation coefficient is given by

$$r_s = 1 - \frac{6 \sum d_i^2}{n^3 - n}$$

where d_i is the difference in the ranks of the two variables for the ith-individual. Alternatively, r_s can be obtained by applying the formula for Pearson's r to the ranks of the variables. The calculation of r_s should be modified when there are tied ranks in the data, but the effect is minimal unless there are many tied ranks.

1 Altman DG, Bland JM. Generalisation and extrapolation. *BMJ* 1998;**317**:409–10.

2 Marre M, Leblanc H, Suarez L, Guyenne T-T, Ménard J, Passa P. Converting enzyme inhibition and kidney function in normotensive diabetic patients with persistent micro-albuminuria. *BMJ* 1987;**294**:1448–52.

3 Armitage P, Berry G. *Statistical methods in medical research.* 3rd edn. Oxford: Blackwell Science, 1994: 336–7.

4 Altman DG. *Practical statistics for medical research.* London: Chapman & Hall, 1991: 336–58.

5 Stubbs P, Collinson P, Moseley D, Greenwood T, Noble M. Prospective study of the role of cardiac troponin T in patients admitted with unstable angina. *BMJ* 1996;**313**:262–4.

6 Møller H, Skakkebæk NE. Risk of testicular cancer in subfertile men: case-control study. *BMJ* 1999;**318**:559–62.

7 Prentice AM, Black AE, Coward WA, *et al.* High levels of energy expenditure in obese women. *BMJ* 1986;**292**:983–7.

9 Time to event studies

DAVID MACHIN, MARTIN J GARDNER

It is common in follow-up studies to be concerned with the survival time between the time of entry to the study and a subsequent event.[1] The event may be death in a study of cancer, the disappearance of pain in a study comparing different steroids in arthritis, or the return of ovulation after stopping a long-acting method of contraception. These studies often generate some so-called "censored" observations of survival time. Such an observation would occur, for example, on any patient who is still alive at the time of analysis in a randomised trial where death is the end point. In this case the time from allocation to treatment to the latest follow-up visit would be the patient's censored survival time.

The Kaplan–Meier product limit technique is the recognised approach for calculating survival curves in such studies.[2,3] An outline of this method is given here. Details of how to calculate a confidence interval for the population value of the survival proportion at any time during the follow up and the median survival are given. Confidence interval calculations are also described for the difference in survival between two groups as expressed by the difference in survival proportions as well as for the hazard ratio between groups which summarises, for example, the relative death or relapse rate.

In some circumstances, the comparison between groups is adjusted for prognostic variables by means of Cox regression.[3] In this case the confidence interval describing the difference between the groups is adjusted for the relevant prognostic variable.

In the survival comparisons context, confidence intervals convey only the effects of sampling variation on the precision of the estimated statistics and cannot control for any non-sampling errors such as bias in the selection of patients or in losses to follow up.

93

Survival proportions

Single sample

Suppose that the survival times after entry to the study (ordered by increasing duration) of a group of n subjects are $t_1, t_2, t_3, \ldots t_n$. The proportion of subjects surviving beyond any follow-up time t, often referred to as $S(t)$ but here denoted p for brevity, is estimated by the Kaplan–Meier technique as

$$p = \prod \frac{r_i - d_i}{r_i},$$

where r_i is the number of subjects alive just before time t_i (the ith ordered survival time), d_i denotes the number who died at time t_i, and $\prod$ indicates multiplication over each time a death occurs up to and including time t.

The standard error (SE) of p is given by

$$\mathrm{SE}(p) = \sqrt{\frac{p(1-p)}{n_{\text{effective}}}},$$

where $n_{\text{effective}}$ is the "effective" sample size at time t. When there are no censored survival times, $n_{\text{effective}}$ will be equal to n, the total number of subjects in the study group. When censored observations are present, the effective sample size is calculated each time a death occurs.[4]

$$n_{\text{effective}} = n - \text{number of subjects censored before time } t.$$

The $100(1 - \alpha)\%$ confidence interval for the population value of the survival proportion p at time t is then calculated as

$$p - [z_{1-\alpha/2} \times \mathrm{SE}(p)] \quad \text{to} \quad p + [z_{1-\alpha/2} \times \mathrm{SE}(p)]$$

where $z_{1-\alpha/2}$ is the appropriate value from the standard Normal distribution for the $100(1 - \alpha/2)$ percentile. Thus for a 95% confidence interval $\alpha = 0.05$ and Table 18.1 gives $z_{1-\alpha/2} = 1.96$.

There are other and more complex alternatives for the calculation of the SE given here including that of Greenwood[5] but, except in situations with very small numbers, these will lead to similar confidence intervals.[3]

The times at which to estimate survival proportions and their confidence intervals should be determined in advance of the results. They can be chosen according to practical convention—for example, the five-year survival proportions which are often quoted in cancer studies—or according to previous similar studies.

Worked example

Consider the survival experience of the 25 patients randomly assigned to receive γ-linolenic acid for the treatment of colorectal cancer of Dukes's stage C.[6] The ordered survival times (t), the calculated survival proportions (p), and the effective sample sizes ($n_{\text{effective}}$) are shown in Table 9.1.

The data come from a comparative trial, but it may be of interest to quote the two-year survival proportion and its confidence interval for the group receiving γ-linolenic acid. The survival proportion to any follow-up time is taken from the entries in the table for that time if

Table 9.1 Survival data by month for 49 patients with Dukes's C colorectal cancer randomly assigned to receive either γ-linolenic acid or control treatment[6]

	Group treated with γ-linolenic acid				Controls		
Patient number	Survival time* (months) (t)	Survival proportion** (p)	Effective sample size[†] ($n_{\text{effective}}$)	Patient number	Survival time* (months) (t)	Survival proportion** (p)	Effective sample size[†] ($n_{\text{effective}}$)
1	1+	1	25	1	3+	1	24
2	5+	1	24	2	6		
3	6			3	6		
4	6	0·9130	23	4	6		
5	9+			5	6	0·8261	23
6	10			6	8		
7	10	0·8217	22	7	8	0·7391	
8	10+			8	12		
9	12			9	12	0·6522	
10	12			10	12+		
11	12			11	15+		22
12	12	0·6284	21	12	16+		21
13	12+			13	18+		
14	13+		20	14	18+		20
15	15+		19	15	20	0·5870	18
16	16+		18	16	22+		
17	20+		17	17	24	0·5136	17
18	24	0·5498	16	18	28+		
19	24+			19	28+		
20	27+		15	20	28+		
21	32	0·4399	14	21	30	0·3852	14
22	34+			22	30+		
23	36+		13	23	33+		13
24	36+			24	42	0	12
25	44+		11				

* Survival times are shown in each group by month to either death or to censoring. Figures with plus signs show that patient follow up was censored.

** Figures need not be recalculated except when a death occurs.

[†] Figures are calculated using method from Peto[4] and need not be recalculated except when a loss to follow up occurs.

available or otherwise for the time immediately preceding. Thus for two years, $t = 24$ months, the survival proportion is $p = S(24) = 0.5498$. The corresponding effective sample size is $n_{\text{effective}} = 16$.

The standard error of this survival proportion is

$$\text{SE}(p) = \sqrt{\frac{0.5498 \times (1 - 0.5498)}{16}} = 0.1244.$$

The 95% confidence interval for the population value of the survival proportion is then given by

$$0.5498 - (1.96 \times 0.1244) \quad \text{to} \quad 0.5498 + (1.96 \times 0.1244)$$

that is, from 0.31 to 0.79.

The estimated percentage of survivors to two years is thus 55% with a 95% confidence interval of 31% to 79%.

Median survival time

Single sample

If there are no censored observations, for example, if all the patients have died on a clinical trial, then the median survival time, M, is estimated by the middle observation (see also chapter 5) of the ordered survival times $t_1, t_2, \ldots, t_n$ if the number of observations n is odd, and by the average of $t_{n/2}$ and $t_{n/2+1}$ if n is even. Thus

$$M = t_{(n+1)/2} \text{ if } n \text{ is odd}$$

or

$$M = \tfrac{1}{2}(t_{n/2} + t_{n/2+1}) \text{ if } n \text{ is even}.$$

Worked example

If we ignore the fact that there are censored observations in Table 9.1 and therefore consider all the patients to have died, then the median survival time of the 25 patients receiving γ-linolenic acid is the 13th ordered observation or $M = 12$ months. Making the same assumption for the 24 patients of the control group the median is the average of the 12th and 13th ordered survival times, that is $M = (16 + 18)/2 = 17$ months.

In the presence of censored survival times the median survival is estimated by first calculating the Kaplan–Meier survival curve, then finding the value of t that satisfies the equation

$$p = S(t) = 0.5.$$

This can be done by extending a horizontal line from $p = 0.5$ (or 50%) on the vertical axis of the Kaplan–Meier survival curve, until the actual curve is met, then moving vertically down from that point to cut the horizontal time axis at $t = M$, which is the estimated median survival time.

The calculations required for the confidence interval of a median are quite complicated and an explanation of how these are derived is complex.[7] The expression for the standard error of the median includes $SE(p)$ described above but evaluated at $p = S(M) = 0.5$. When $p = 0.5$,

$$SE(p) = \sqrt{\frac{0.5 \times 0.5}{n_{\text{effective}}}} = \frac{0.5}{\sqrt{n_{\text{effective}}}}.$$

The standard error of the median is given by

$$SE(M) = \frac{0.5}{\sqrt{n_{\text{effective}}}} \times [(t_{\text{small}} - t_{\text{large}})/(p_{\text{large}} - p_{\text{small}})],$$

where t_{small} is the smallest observed survival time from the Kaplan–Meier curve for which p is less than or equal to 0.45, while t_{large} is the largest observed survival time from the Kaplan–Meier curve for which p is greater than 0.55. The ratio $[(t_{\text{small}} - t_{\text{large}})/(p_{\text{large}} - p_{\text{small}})]$ in the above expression, estimates the height of the distribution of survival times at the median. Just as the blood pressure values of chapter 4 have a distribution, in that case taking the Normal distribution form, survival times will also have an underlying distribution of some form. The values of 0.45 and 0.55 are chosen at each side of the median of 0.5 to define "small" and "large" and are arbitrary. Should $p_{\text{large}} = p_{\text{small}}$ then the two values will need to be chosen wider apart. They may be chosen closer to 0.5 for large study sizes.

The $100(1 - \alpha)\%$ confidence interval for the population value of the median survival M is then calculated as

$$M - [z_{1-\alpha/2} \times SE(M)] \quad \text{to} \quad M + [z_{1-\alpha/2} \times SE(M)],$$

where $z_{1-\alpha/2}$ is obtained from Table 18.1.

However, we must caution against the uncritical use of this method for small data sets as the value of $SE(M)$ is unreliable in such circumstances, and also the values of t_{small} and t_{large} will be poorly determined.

Worked example

The Kaplan–Meier survival curve for the control patients of Table 9.1 is shown in Figure 9.1 and the hatched line indicates how the median is

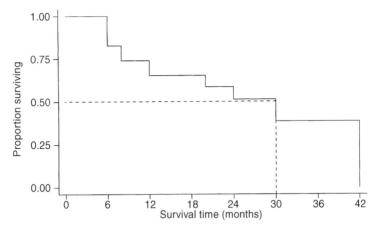

Figure 9.1 Kaplan–Meier estimate of the survival curve of 24 patients with Dukes's C colorectal cancer.[6]

estimated. This gives $M = 30$ months. (We note that this is quite different from the *incorrect* value given in the illustrative example above.)

The effective sample size at 30 months is $n_{\text{effective}} = 14$ so that

$$\text{SE}(M) = \frac{0{\cdot}5}{\sqrt{14}} = 0{\cdot}1336.$$

Reading from Table 9.1 at $p_{\text{small}} = 0{\cdot}3852 < 0{\cdot}45$ gives $t_{\text{small}} = 30$ months also, and for $p_{\text{large}} = 0{\cdot}5870 > 0{\cdot}55$ gives $t_{\text{large}} = 20$ months.

Thus

$$\text{SE}(M) = 0{\cdot}1336 \times \frac{(30 - 20)}{(0{\cdot}5870 - 0{\cdot}3852)} = 6{\cdot}6230.$$

The 95% confidence interval is therefore

$$30 - (1{\cdot}96 \times 6{\cdot}6230) \quad \text{to} \quad 30 + (1{\cdot}96 \times 6{\cdot}6230),$$

that is, from $17{\cdot}0$ to $43{\cdot}0$ months.

The estimated median survival is 30 months with a 95% confidence interval of 17 to 43 months. For the γ-linolenic acid group $M = 32$ months and $\text{SE}(M) = 14{\cdot}18$.

Two samples

The difference between survival proportions at any time t in two study groups of sample sizes n_1 and n_2 is measured by $p_1 - p_2$, where $p_1 = S_1(t)$ and $p_2 = S_2(t)$ are the survival proportions at time t in groups 1 and 2 respectively.

The standard error of $p_1 - p_2$ is

$$SE(p_1 - p_2) = \sqrt{\frac{p_1(1 - p_1)}{n_{\text{effective},1}} + \frac{p_2(1 - p_2)}{n_{\text{effective},2}}}$$

where $n_{\text{effective},1}$ and $n_{\text{effective},2}$ are the effective sample sizes at time t in each group.

The $100(1 - \alpha)\%$ confidence interval for the population value of $p_1 - p_2$ is

$$p_1 - p_2 - [z_{1-\alpha/2} \times SE(p_1 - p_2)] \quad \text{to}$$

$$p_1 - p_2 + [z_{1-\alpha/2} \times SE(p_1 - p_2)],$$

where $z_{1-\alpha/2}$ is obtained from Table 18.1.

Worked example

The survival experience of the patients receiving γ-linolenic acid and the controls can be compared from the results given in Table 9.1. At two years for example, $p_1 = 0.5498$ and $p_2 = 0.5136$ with $n_{\text{effctive},1} = 16$ and $n_{\text{effective},2} = 17$. The estimated difference in two-year survival proportions is thus $0.5498 - 0.5136 = 0.0363$.

The standard error of this difference in survival proportions is

$$\sqrt{\frac{0.5498(1 - 0.5498)}{16} + \frac{0.5136(1 - 0.5136)}{17}} = 0.1737.$$

The 95% confidence interval for the population value of the difference in two-year survival proportions is then given by

$$0.0363 - (1.96 \times 0.1737) \quad \text{to} \quad 0.0363 + (1.96 \times 0.1737)$$

that is, from -0.30 to 0.38.

Thus the study estimate of the increased survival proportion at two years for the patients given γ-linolenic acid compared with the control group is only about 4%. Moreover, the imprecision in the estimate from this small study is indicated by the 95% confidence interval ranging from -30% to $+38\%$.

Difference between median survival times

The difference between the median survival times in two study groups of sample sizes n_1 and n_2 is measured by $M_1 - M_2$, where M_1 and M_2 are the medians in groups 1 and 2 respectively. The standard error of $M_1 - M_2$ is

$$SE(M_1 - M_2) = \sqrt{[(SE(M_1)]^2 + [SE(M_2)]^2}.$$

The $100(1 - \alpha)\%$ confidence interval for the population value of $M_1 - M_2$ is

$$M_1 - M_2 - [z_{1-\alpha/2} \times \text{SE}(M_1 - M_2)] \quad \text{to}$$

$$M_1 - M_2 + [z_{1-\alpha/2} \times \text{SE}(M_1 - M_2)],$$

where $z_{1-\alpha/2}$ is obtained from Table 18.1.

Worked example

The median survival experiences of the patients receiving γ-linolenic acid and the controls can be compared from the results given in Table 9.1. Thus $M_1 = 32$ and $M_2 = 30$ months, a difference of $M_1 - M_2 = 2$ months. The standard error of this difference is estimated by

$$\sqrt{(14 \cdot 1783)^2 + (6 \cdot 6230)^2} = 15 \cdot 65.$$

The 95% confidence interval for the population value of the difference in medians is then given by

$$2 - (1 \cdot 96 \times 15 \cdot 65) \quad \text{to} \quad 2 + (1 \cdot 96 \times 15 \cdot 65)$$

that is, from $-28 \cdot 7$ to $32 \cdot 7$ months.

Thus the study estimate of the increased median survival for the patients given γ-linolenic acid compared with the control group is only 2 months. Moreover, the imprecision in the estimate from this small study is indicated by the 95% confidence interval ranging from -29 to $+33$ months.

The hazard ratio

In a follow-up study of two groups the ratio of failure rates—for example, death or relapse rates—is termed the "hazard ratio". It is a common measure of the relative effect of treatments or exposures. If O_1 and O_2 are the total numbers of deaths observed in the two groups then the corresponding expected numbers of deaths (E_1 and E_2), assuming an equal risk of dying at each time in both groups, may be calculated as

$$E_1 = \sum \frac{r_{1i}d_i}{r_i} \quad \text{and} \quad E_2 = \sum \frac{r_{2i}d_i}{r_i}.$$

Here r_{1i} and r_{2i} are the numbers of subjects alive and not censored in groups 1 and 2 just before time t_i with $r_i = r_{1i} + r_{2i}$; $d_i = d_{1i} + d_{2i}$ is the number who died at time t_i in the two groups combined; and $\sum$ indicates addition over each time of death.

100

One estimator of the hazard ratio (HR) is $(O_1/E_1)/(O_2/E_2)$ although, for technical reasons, the more complex estimator

$$HR = \exp\left(\frac{O_1 - E_1}{V}\right),$$

where

$$V = \sum \frac{r_{1i}r_{2i}d_i(r_i - d_i)}{r_i^2(r_i - 1)},$$

is more appropriate.

To obtain a $100(1 - \alpha)\%$ confidence interval for the population value of the hazard ratio one first calculates the two quantities

$$X = \frac{O_1 - E_1}{V} \quad \text{and} \quad Y = \frac{z_{1-\alpha/2}}{\sqrt{V}},$$

where $z_{1-\alpha/2}$ is the appropriate value from the standard Normal distribution for the $100(1 - \alpha/2)$ percentile (see Table 18.1). Thus for a 95% confidence interval $\alpha = 0.05$ and $z_{1-\alpha/2} = 1.96$.

The hazard ratio can then be estimated by HR and the confidence interval for the hazard ratio by[8]

$$e^{X - Y} \quad \text{to} \quad e^{X + Y}.$$

The hazard ratio calculated from $(O_1/E_1)/(O_2/E_2)$ will be close to e^X except in unusual data sets.

Worked example

For the data at the end of the trial, shown in Table 9.1, $O_1 = 10$, $E_1 = 11.37$, $O_2 = 12$, $E_2 = 10.63$, and $V = 4.99$.

The values of X and for Y, with $\alpha = 0.05$, are

$$X = \frac{10 - 11.37}{4.99} = -0.28 \quad \text{and} \quad Y = \frac{1.96}{\sqrt{4.99}} = 0.88.$$

The hazard ratio is thus estimated as

$$HR = e^{-0.28} = 0.76.$$

The 95% confidence interval for the population value of the hazard ratio is then given by

$$e^{-1.15} \quad \text{to} \quad e^{0.60},$$

that is, from 0.32 to 1.83.

The results indicate that treatment with γ-linolenic acid has been associated with an estimated reduction in mortality to 76% of that for the control treatment, while the alternative hazard ratio calculation gives a similar figure of 78%. The reduction, however, is imprecisely estimated as shown by the wide confidence interval of 32% to 183%.

In the case when the distributions for the two groups can be assumed to be from exponential distributions, the ratio of the inverse of the two medians provides an estimate of the hazard ratio, that is, $HR_{\text{median}} = M_2/M_1$. In this case, the approximate confidence interval is given as[9]

$$\frac{M_2}{M_1} - e^{-z_{1-\alpha/2} \times \text{SE}(HR_{\text{median}})} \quad \text{to} \quad \frac{M_2}{M_1} + e^{-z_{1-\alpha/2} \times \text{SE}(HR_{\text{median}})}$$

where

$$\text{SE}(HR_{\text{median}}) = \sqrt{\frac{1}{O_1} + \frac{1}{O_2}}.$$

As noted earlier, O_1 and O_2 are the number of deaths in the respective groups.

Worked example

For the data at the end of the study, shown in Table 9.1, $M_1 = 32$, $M_2 = 30$, while $O_1 = 10$ and $O_2 = 12$. This gives an estimate of the hazard ratio as $30/32 = 0.9375$. This is equivalent to a reduction in mortality of 6%. The corresponding standard error is

$$\text{SE}(HR_{\text{median}}) = \sqrt{\frac{1}{10} + \frac{1}{12}} = 0.4282.$$

The 95% confidence interval for the population value of the hazard ratio is then given by

$$0.9375 - e^{(-1.96 \times 0.4282)} \quad \text{to} \quad 0.9375 + e^{(-1.96 \times 0.4282)},$$

that is, from $0.9375 - 0.4320$ to $0.9375 + 0.4320$, or 0.51 to 1.37.

Cox regression

Just as in the situations described in chapter 8 in which the linear regression equation is used for predicting one variable from another, it is often important to relate the outcome measure (here survival time) to other variables. In contrast to the y variable of chapter 8, the comparable variable is time t but with the added complication that this will usually have censored values in some cases. As a consequence, and for quite technical reasons, special methods have been developed for survival time regression.[10] These Cox regression models are then utilised in much the same way as the regression models of chapter 8. In the special case of a comparison between two groups of subjects, the Cox model provides essentially the same estimate of *HR* and the associated confidence interval as described earlier. The basic assumption is that the risk of failure (death) in one group is the same constant multiple of the other group at any point in the follow-up time.[3]

The Cox regression model for the comparison of two groups assumes that the risk of death in the two groups can be respectively described by

$$\lambda_1(t) = \lambda_0(t)e^{\beta x_1} \quad \text{and} \quad \lambda_2(t) = \lambda_0(t)e^{\beta x_2}.$$

Here if $\beta = 0$ then both groups have the same underlying death rate (hazard), $\lambda_0(t)$, at each time t, but this rate may change over time. For comparing two groups, it is usual to write $x_1 = 1$ and $x_2 = 0$, in which case

$$HR_{\text{Cox}} = \frac{\lambda_1(t)}{\lambda_2(t)} = \frac{\lambda_0(t)e^{\beta}}{\lambda_0(t)} = e^{\beta}.$$

Since t does not appear in the above expression (e^{β}) the hazard ratio does not change with time.

The $100(1 - \alpha)\%$ confidence interval for the population hazard ratio is

$$e^{[\beta - z_{1-\alpha/2} \times \text{SE}(\beta)]} \quad \text{to} \quad e^{[\beta + z_{1-\alpha/2} \times \text{SE}(\beta)]}$$

where $\text{SE}(\beta)$ is obtained from a computer program.

Worked example

For the data of Table 9.1 use of a standard statistical package gives $\beta = -0.2528$, with $\text{SE}(\beta) = 0.4302$. Thus the $HR_{\text{Cox}} = e^{-0.2528} = 0.78$. The corresponding 95% confidence interval for the hazard ratio is

$$e^{(-0.2528 - 1.96 \times 0.4302)} = e^{-1.0960} \quad \text{to} \quad e^{(-0.2528 + 1.96 \times 0.4302)} = e^{0.5900}$$

or 0.33 to 1.80.

It is useful to note that the estimate of HR_{Cox} and the corresponding 95% confidence interval are similar to those given in earlier calculations. They differ somewhat from those corresponding to HR_{median} for which the assumption of a constant hazard (one that does not change with t) was made within each treatment group.

In certain circumstances there may be prognostic features of individual patients which may influence their survival and thus may modify the observed difference between groups. In such cases, we wish to compare the groups taking account of (or adjusted for) these variables. This leads to extending the single-variable Cox model just described (with one explanatory variable indicating the group) to include also one or more prognostic variables as one may do in other multiple regression situations (see chapter 8). In the context of randomised controlled trials, described in chapter 11, we wish to check whether or not the treatment effect observed, as expressed by the hazard ratio, will be modified after taking account of these prognostic variables.[3]

1 Bland JM, Altman DG. Time to event (survival) data. *BMJ* 1997;**317**:468–9.
2 Altman DG, Bland JM. Survival probabilities (the Kaplan–Meier method). *BMJ* 1997;**317**:1572.
3 Parmar MKB, Machin D. *Survival analysis: a practical approach.* Chichester: John Wiley, 1995:26–40;115–42.
4 Peto J. The calculation and interpretation of survival curves. In: Buyse ME, Staquet MJ, Sylvester RJ (eds). *Cancer clinical trials: methods and practice.* Oxford: Oxford University Press, 1984:361–80.
5 Greenwood M. *The natural duration of cancer.* Reports of Public Health and Medical Subjects, 33. London: HMSO, 1926.
6 McIllmurray MB, Turkie W. Controlled trial of γ-linolenic acid in Dukes's C colorectal cancer. *BMJ* 1987;**294**:1260 and **295**:475.
7 Collett D. *Modelling survival data in medical research.* London: Chapman & Hall, 1994: section 2·4.
8 Daly L. Confidence intervals. *BMJ* 1988;**297**:66.
9 Altman DG. *Practical statistics for medical research.* London: Chapman & Hall, 1991:384–5.
10 Cox DR. Regression models and life tables (with discussion). *J R Statist Soc Ser B* 1972;**34**:187–220.

10 Diagnostic tests

DOUGLAS G ALTMAN

Studies evaluating diagnostic test performance yield a variety of numerical results. While these ought to be accompanied by confidence intervals, this is less commonly done than in other types of medical research.[1]

Diagnosis may be based either on the presence or absence of some feature or symptom, on a classification into three or more groups (perhaps using a pathological grading system), or on a measurement. Values of a measurement may also be grouped into two or more categories, or may be kept as measurements. Each case will be considered in turn. See Altman[2] for more detailed discussion of most of these methods.

A confidence interval indicates uncertainty in the estimated value. As noted in earlier chapters, it does not take account of any additional uncertainty that might relate to other aspects such as bias in the study design, a common problem with studies evaluating diagnostic studies.[3]

Classification into two groups

Sensitivity and specificity

The simplest diagnostic test is one where the results of an investigation, such as an X-ray or biopsy, are used to classify patients into two groups according to the presence or absence of a symptom or sign. The question is then to quantify the ability of this binary test to discriminate between patients who do or do not have the disease or condition of interest. (The general term "disease" is used here, although the target disorder is not always a disease.) Table 10.1 shows a 2×2 table representing this situation, in which a, b, c, and d are the numbers of individuals in each cell of the table.

Table 10.1 Relation between a binary diagnostic test and presence or absence of disease

		Disease		Total
		+	−	
Test	+	True +ve a	False +ve b	$a + b$
	−	False −ve c	True −ve d	$c + d$
	Total	$a + c$	$b + d$	n

The two most common indices of the performance of a test are the sensitivity and specificity. The *sensitivity* is the proportion of true positives that are correctly identified by the test, given by $a/(a + c)$ in Table 10.1. The *specificity* is the proportion of true negatives that are correctly identified by the test, or $d/(b + d)$.

The sensitivity and specificity are proportions, and so confidence intervals can be calculated for them using the traditional method or Wilson's method, as discussed in chapter 6. Note that the traditional method may not perform well when proportions are close to 1 (100%) as is often the case in this context, and may even give confidence intervals which exceed 100%.[4] Wilson's method is thus generally preferable.

Worked example

Petersen *et al.*[5] investigated the use of the ice-water test in 80 patients with detrusor overactivity. Of these, 60 had bladder instability and 20 had detrusor hyperreflexia. Their results are shown in Table 10.2.

The sensitivity of the test at detecting detrusor hyperreflexia was $39/60 = 0.650$ or 65.0% and the specificity was $17/20 = 0.850$ or

Table 10.2 Results of ice-water test among patients with either detrusor hyperreflexia (DH) or bladder instability (BI)[5]

		DH (+)	BI (−)	Total
	+	True +ve 39	False +ve 3	42
Test	−	False −ve 21	True −ve 17	38
	Total	60	20	80

85·0%. Using the recommended method (Wilson's method), 95% confidence intervals are 52·4% to 75·8% for the sensitivity and 64·0% to 94·8% for the specificity.

The traditional method gives a similar confidence interval for the sensitivity of 52·9% to 75·8%, but an impossible confidence interval for the specificity of 69·4% to 100·6%.

Positive and negative predictive values

In clinical practice the test result is all that is known, so we want to know how good the test is at predicting abnormality. In other words, what proportion of patients with abnormal test results are truly abnormal? The sensitivity and specificity do not give us this information. Instead we must approach the data from the direction of the test results. These two proportions are defined as follows:

- *Positive predictive value* (*PV+*) is the proportion of patients with positive test results who are correctly diagnosed.
- *Negative predictive value* (*PV−*) is the proportion of patients with negative test results who are correctly diagnosed.

In the notation of Table 10.1, $PV+ = a/(a+b)$ and $PV- = d/(c+d)$.

Worked example

Using the same data as before, the positive predictive value among those with a positive ice-water test is $PV+ = 39/42$ (92·9%) and the negative predictive value among those with a negative test result is $PV- = 17/38$ (44·7%). Using Wilson's method (chapter 6), 95% confidence intervals are 81·0% to 97·5% for the positive predictive value and 30·1 % to 60·3% for the negative predictive value.

We should not stop the analysis here. The predictive values of a test depend upon the prevalence of the abnormality in the patients being tested, which may not be known. The values just calculated assume that the prevalence of detrusor hyperreflexia among the population of patients likely to be tested is the same as in the sample, namely 60/80 or 75%. In a different clinical setting the prevalence of abnormality may differ considerably.

Predictive values observed in one study do not apply universally. The rarer the true abnormality is, the more sure we can be that a negative test indicates no abnormality, and the less sure that a positive result really indicates an abnormal patient.

More general formulae for calculating predictive values for any prevalence (*prev*) are

$$PV+ = \frac{sens \times prev}{(sens \times prev) + (1 - spec) \times (1 - prev)}$$

and

$$PV- = \frac{spec \times (1 - prev)}{(1 - sens) \times prev + spec \times (1 - prev)},$$

where *sens* and *spec* are the sensitivity and specificity as previously defined. The prevalence can be interpreted as the probability before the test is carried out that the subject has the disease, also known as the prior probability of disease. $PV+$ and $PV-$ are the revised estimates of the probability of disease for those subjects who are positive and negative to the test, and are known as *posterior probabilities*. The comparison of the prior and posterior probabilities is one way of assessing the usefulness of the test. The predictive values can change considerably with a different prevalence.

We can obtain approximate confidence intervals for prevalence-adjusted predictive values by expressing them as proportions of the number of positive or negative test results in the study.

Worked example

We can estimate the predictive values for a setting where the prevalence of detrusor hyperreflexia is 25% (0·25). For example, the prevalence-adjusted positive predicted value is

$$PV+ = \frac{0·65 \times 0·25}{(0·65 \times 0·25) + (1 - 0·85) \times (1 - 0·25)}$$

$$= 0·591 \quad \text{or} \quad 59·1\%.$$

With the estimated prevalence-adjusted $PV+$ of 0·591, in a sample of 42 test positives we would expect $0·591 \times 42 = 24·8$ true positives, or about 25. We can construct a confidence interval for the proportion 25/42 in the usual way. Wilson's method gives a 95% confidence interval around the adjusted $PV+$ of 0·591 from 0·445 to 0·730, or 44·5% to 73·0%.

Likelihood ratios

For any test result we can compare the probability of getting that result, if the patient truly had the condition of interest, with the corresponding probability if they were healthy. The ratio of these probabilities is called the likelihood ratio (LR). The likelihood ratio for a positive test result is calculated as

$$LR+ = sens/(1 - spec)$$

and the likelihood ratio for a negative test result is calculated as

$$LR- = (1 - sens)/spec.$$

The contrast between these values indicates the value of the test for increasing certainty about a diagnosis.[2]

Worked example

Using the same data as before, the prevalence of detrusor hyperreflexia was 0·75. The likelihood ratio for a positive test is $LR+ = 0·65/(1 - 0·85) = 4·33$ and the likelihood ratio for a negative test is $LR- = (1 - 0·65)/0·85 = 0·41$.

The likelihood ratio is increasingly being quoted in papers describing diagnostic test results, but is rarely accompanied by a confidence interval. The likelihood ratio for a positive test can be also expressed as the ratio of the true-positive and false-positive rates, that is

$$LR+ = \frac{a/(a+c)}{b/(b+d)}.$$

Similarly, the likelihood ratio for a negative test can be expressed as the ratio of the true-negative and false-negative rates, that is

$$LR- = \frac{d/(b+d)}{c/(a+c)}.$$

The likelihood ratio is identical in construction to a relative risk (or risk ratio)—that is, it is the ratio of two independent proportions. It follows immediately that a method for deriving a confidence interval for a relative risk can be applied also to the likelihood ratio. There are several possible methods, not all of which are equally good. Two are considered here.

Log method

Confidence intervals for the population value of the likelihood ratio can be constructed through a logarithmic transformation,[2] as described in chapter 7. The method is illustrated using LR+. The standard error of $\log_e LR+$ is

$$SE(\log_e LR+) = \sqrt{\frac{1}{a} - \frac{1}{a+c} + \frac{1}{b} - \frac{1}{b+d}}$$

from which a $100(1 - \alpha)\%$ confidence interval for $\log_e LR+$ is found in the standard way. We obtain a confidence interval for $LR+$ by antilogging (exponentiating) these values. (The derivation of this method, sometimes called the log method, is given in the appendix of Simel et al.[6])

Note that either a or b can be zero, in which case $SE(\log_e LR+)$ becomes infinite. To avoid this problem, it may be preferable in such cases to add 0·5 to the counts in all four cells of the observed table before calculating both $LR+$ and $SE(\log_e LR+)$.

Score method

The "score test" method reportedly performs somewhat better that the usual log method,[7,8] although it is too complex for the formula to be given here.

Worked example

Nam[8] (1995) considered the following example, originally provided by Koopman:[9] 36/40 diseased and 16/80 non-diseased patients have positive test results. We thus have $a = 36, b = 16, c = 4$, and $d = 64$. The estimated likelihood ratio for a positive test is $LR+ = (36/40)/(16/80) = 4.5$. The log method gives a 95% confidence interval for $LR+$ from 2·87 to 7·06. Using the score method, the 95% confidence interval is 2·94 to 7·15, so in this case the two methods agree reasonably well.

Classification into more than two groups

Multicategory classifications represent an intermediate step between dichotomous tests and tests based on measurements. With few categories, say three or four, we can evaluate the preceding statistics using in turn each division between categories to create a binary test. Sometimes this procedure is adopted for tests which are measurements. For example, Sackett et al.[10] discuss the use of serum ferritin level in five bands to diagnose, or rule out, iron-deficiency anaemia.

Diagnostic tests based on measurements

Many diagnostic tests are quantitative, notably in clinical chemistry. The methods of the preceding sections can be applied only if we can select a cutpoint to distinguish "normal" from "abnormal", which is not a trivial problem. It is often done by taking the observed median value, or perhaps the upper limit of a predetermined reference interval.

This approach is wasteful of information, however, and involves a degree of arbitrariness. Classification into several groups is better than just two, but there are ways of proceeding that do not require any grouping of the data; they are described in this section.

The area under a receiver operating characteristic (ROC) curve

First we can investigate to what extent the test results differ among people who do or do not have the diagnosis of interest. The receiver operating characteristic (ROC) plot is one way to do this. ROC plots were developed in the 1950s for evaluating radar signal detection. A paper by Hanley and McNeil[11] was very influential in introducing the method to medicine.

The ROC plot is obtained by calculating the sensitivity and specificity for every distinct observed data value and plotting sensitivity against 1 – specificity, as in Figure 10.1. A test that discriminates perfectly between the two groups would yield a

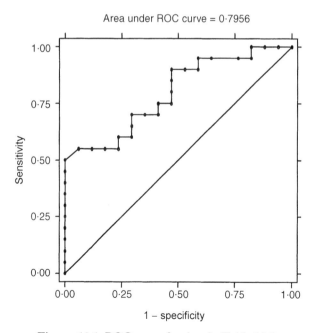

Figure 10.1 ROC curve for data in Table 10.3.

111

"curve" that coincided with the left and top sides of the plot. A test that is completely useless would give a straight line from the bottom left corner to the top right corner. In practice the ROC curve will lie somewhere between these extremes according to the degree of overlap of the values in the groups.

A global assessment of the performance of the test, sometimes called diagnostic accuracy,[12] is given by the area under the ROC curve (often abbreviated AUC). This area is equal to the probability that a random person with the disease has a higher value of the measurement than a random person without the disease. The area is 1 for a perfect test and 0·5 for an uninformative test. The nonparametric calculation of the area under the curve is closely related to the Mann–Whitney U statistic.

The area under the curve and its standard error can be obtained by examining every comparison of a member of each group. We consider the n individuals in the first group with values X_i and the m individuals in the second group with observations Y_j, so that there are nm pairs of values X_i and Y_j. For each pair we obtain a "placement score" ψ_{ij}, which indicates which value is larger. We have $\psi_{ij} = 1$ if $Y_j > X_i$; $\psi_{ij} = 0·5$ if $Y_j = X_i$; and $\psi_{ij} = 0$ if $Y_j < X_i$. In effect we assess where each observation is placed compared with all of the values in the other group.[14,15] The area under the curve is simply the mean of all of the values ψ_{ij}. In mathematical notation, we have

$$AUC = \frac{1}{nm} \sum_{i=1}^{n} \sum_{j=1}^{m} \psi_{ij}.$$

The area under the curve can also be written as

$$AUC = \frac{1}{nm} \sum_{i=1}^{n} R_i = \frac{1}{nm} \sum_{j=1}^{m} C_j$$

where

$$R_i = \sum_{j=1}^{m} \psi_{ij} \quad \text{and} \quad C_j = \sum_{i=1}^{n} \psi_{ij}.$$

The values R_i indicate for each member of the first group the proportion of the observations in the second group which exceed it, and similarly for C_j. (They are also the row and column totals of ψ_{ij} when the data are arranged in a two-way table, as in the worked example below.)

To get the standard error of AUC we first calculate the quantities

$$S_X^2 = \frac{1}{n-1} \sum_{i=1}^{n} \left(\frac{R_i}{m} - AUC \right)^2$$

and

$$S_Y^2 = \frac{1}{m-1} \sum_{j=1}^{m} \left(\frac{C_j}{n} - AUC \right)^2.$$

The standard error of AUC is then given by

$$\text{SE}(AUC) = \sqrt{\frac{S_X^2}{n} + \frac{S_Y^2}{m}}.$$

An equivalent method, based on the values of R_i and C_j, and avoiding the need to calculate S_X^2 and S_Y^2, is

$$\text{SE}(AUC) = \sqrt{\frac{1}{nm} [\text{var}(R_i) + \text{var}(C_j)]}$$

where var indicates the variance. The standard error of AUC, the area under the ROC curve, can be used to construct a confidence interval in the familiar way using the general formula given in chapter 3. A $100(1 - \alpha)\%$ confidence interval for AUC is

$$AUC - z_{1-\alpha/2} \times \text{SE}(AUC) \quad \text{to} \quad AUC + z_{1-\alpha/2} \times \text{SE}(AUC)$$

where $z_{1-\alpha/2}$ is the appropriate value from the standard Normal distribution for the $100(1 - \alpha/2)$ percentile (see Table 18.1). For a 95% confidence interval, $z_{1-\alpha/2} = 1.96$.

Worked example

Table 10.3 shows values of an index of mixed epidermal cell lymphocyte reactions in bone-marrow transplant recipients who did or did not develop graft-versus-host disease (GvHD).[13] The usefulness of the test for predicting GvHD is related to the degree of non-overlap in the two distributions. The ROC curve for these data is shown in Figure 10.1. Table 10.4 shows the values of ψ_{ij} for each combination of one member of each group, where the X_i are the observations from 17 patients with GvHD and Y_j are the values from the 20 patients without GvHD.

The area under the curve is obtained simply as the mean of the entries in Table 10.4, given by $AUC = 270.5/(17 \times 20) = 0.7956$, or about 0.8, showing quite good separation between the groups.

Table 10.3 Values of an index of mixed epidermal cell lymphocyte reactions in bone-marrow transplant recipients who did or did not develop graft-versus-host disease (GvHD)[13]

With GvHD ($n = 17$)		Without GvHD ($m = 20$)	
1·10	4·13	0·27	1·10
1·16	4·52	0·31	1·52
1·45	4·52	0·39	1·88
1·50	4·71	0·48	2·01
1·85	5·07	0·49	2·40
2·30	9·00	0·50	2·45
2·34	10·11	0·81	2·60
2·44		0·82	2·64
3·70		0·86	3·78
3·73		0·92	4·72

The variances of the row and column totals are 4·3633 and 3·7259 respectively, so that

$$\mathrm{SE}(AUC) = \sqrt{\frac{1}{340}\left(\frac{4\cdot3633^2}{17} + \frac{3\cdot7259^2}{20}\right)} = 0\cdot0730.$$

The 95% confidence interval for the area under the curve is thus $0\cdot7956 - 1\cdot96 \times 0\cdot0730$ to $0\cdot7956 + 1\cdot96 \times 0\cdot0730$, that is 0·65 to 0·94. The confidence interval is quite wide because the sample size is small.

The method just described relies on the assumption that the area under the curve has a Normal sampling distribution. Obuchowski and Lieber[16] note that for methods of high accuracy ($AUC > 0\cdot95$) use of the preceding method for the area under a single ROC curve may require a sample size of 200. For smaller samples a bootstrap approach is recommended (see chapter 13).

Having determined that a test does provide good discrimination the choice can be made of the best cutpoint for clinical use. The simple approach of minimising "errors" (equivalent to maximising the sum of the sensitivity and specificity) is common, but it is not necessarily best. Consideration needs to be given to the costs (not just financial) of false-negative and false-positive diagnoses, and the prevalence of the disease in the subjects being tested.[12] For example, when screening the general population for cancer the cutpoint would be chosen to ensure that most cases were detected (high sensitivity) at the cost of many false positives (low specificity), who could be eliminated by a further test.

Table 10.4 Placement scores (ψ_{ij}) for the data in Table 10.3

	1·10	1·16	1·45	1·50	1·85	2·30	2·34	2·44	3·70	3·73	4·13	4·52	4·52	4·71	5·07	9·00	10·11	Total
0·27	1	1	1	1	1	1	1	1	1	1	1	1	1	1	1	1	1	17
0·31	1	1	1	1	1	1	1	1	1	1	1	1	1	1	1	1	1	17
0·39	1	1	1	1	1	1	1	1	1	1	1	1	1	1	1	1	1	17
0·48	1	1	1	1	1	1	1	1	1	1	1	1	1	1	1	1	1	17
0·49	1	1	1	1	1	1	1	1	1	1	1	1	1	1	1	1	1	17
0·50	1	1	1	1	1	1	1	1	1	1	1	1	1	1	1	1	1	17
0·81	1	1	1	1	1	1	1	1	1	1	1	1	1	1	1	1	1	17
0·82	1	1	1	1	1	1	1	1	1	1	1	1	1	1	1	1	1	17
0·86	1	1	1	1	1	1	1	1	1	1	1	1	1	1	1	1	1	17
0·92	1	1	1	1	1	1	1	1	1	1	1	1	1	1	1	1	1	17
1·10	½	1	1	1	1	1	1	1	1	1	1	1	1	1	1	1	1	16·5
1·52	0	0	0	0	1	1	1	1	1	1	1	1	1	1	1	1	1	13
1·88	0	0	0	0	0	1	1	1	1	1	1	1	1	1	1	1	1	12
2·01	0	0	0	0	0	1	1	1	1	1	1	1	1	1	1	1	1	12
2·40	0	0	0	0	0	0	0	1	1	1	1	1	1	1	1	1	1	10
2·45	0	0	0	0	0	0	0	0	1	1	1	1	1	1	1	1	1	9
2·60	0	0	0	0	0	0	0	0	1	1	1	1	1	1	1	1	1	9
2·64	0	0	0	0	0	0	0	0	1	1	1	1	1	1	1	1	1	9
3·78	0	0	0	0	0	0	0	0	0	0	1	1	1	1	1	1	1	7
4·72	0	0	0	0	0	0	0	0	0	0	0	0	0	0	1	1	1	3
Total	10·5	11	11	11	12	14	14	15	18	18	19	19	19	19	20	20	20	270·5

The ROC plot is more useful when comparing two or more measures. A test with a curve that lies wholly above the curve of another will be clearly better. Methods for comparing the areas under two ROC curves for both paired and unpaired data are reviewed by Zweig and Campbell.[12]

Comparison of assessors—the kappa statistic

An important aspect of classifying patients into two or more categories is the consistency with which it can be done. Of particular interest here is the ability of different observers to agree on the classification. A similar situation arises when we wish to compare two alternative diagnostic tests to see how well they agree with each other. In each case, we can construct a two-way table such as Table 10.5 and compare the observed agreement with that which we would expect by chance alone, using the statistic known as kappa (κ).

Kappa is a measure of agreement beyond the level of agreement expected by chance alone. The observed agreement is the proportion of samples for which both observers agree, given by $p_o = (a + d)/n$. To get the expected agreement we use the row and column totals to estimate the expected numbers agreeing for each category. For positive agreement $(+, +)$ the expected proportion is the product of $(a + b)/n$ and $(a + c)/n$, giving $(a + b)(a + c)/n^2$. Likewise, for negative agreement the expected proportion is $(c + d)(b + d)/n^2$. The expected proportion of agreements for the whole table (p_e) is the sum of these two terms. From these elements we obtain kappa as

$$\kappa = \frac{p_o - p_e}{1 - p_e}$$

Table 10.5 Comparison of binary assessments by two observers

		Observer 1		
		$+$	$-$	Total
Observer 2	$+$	a	b	$a + b$
	$-$	c	d	$c + d$
	Total	$a + c$	$b + d$	n

and its standard error is

$$\mathrm{SE}(\kappa) = \sqrt{\frac{p_\mathrm{o}(1 - p_\mathrm{o})}{n(1 - p_\mathrm{e})^2}},$$

from which a $100(1 - \alpha)\%$ confidence interval for κ is found in the standard way as

$$\kappa - z_{1 - \alpha/2} \times \mathrm{SE}(\kappa) \quad \mathrm{to} \quad \kappa + z_{1 - \alpha/2} \times \mathrm{SE}(\kappa)$$

where $z_{1 - \alpha/2}$ is defined as above.

Kappa has its maximum value of 1 when there is perfect agreement. A kappa value of 0 indicates agreement no better than chance, while negative values (rarely encountered) indicate agreement worse than chance.

Worked example

A group of children who had survived post-haemorrhagic ventricular dilatation were assessed by a paediatrician and by their parents regarding their ability to perform various activities. Table 10.6 shows the relation between their assessments of whether the child could walk downstairs. The observed agreement is $p_\mathrm{o} = (32 + 42)/83 = 0.8916$. The expected agreement is $p_\mathrm{e} = (35 \times 38)/83^2 + (48 \times 45)/83^2 = 0.5066$. From these we calculate kappa as

$$\kappa = \frac{0.8916 - 0.5066}{1 - 0.5066} = 0.780.$$

The standard error of kappa is

$$\mathrm{SE}(\kappa) = \sqrt{\frac{0.8916 \times (1 - 0.8916)}{83 \times (1 - 0.5066)^2}} = 0.0692.$$

Table 10.6 Comparison of paediatrician's and parent's assessments of whether children could walk downstairs[17]

| | | Paediatrician | | Total |
		Yes	No	
Parent	Yes	32	6	38
	No	3	42	45
	Total	35	48	83

The 95% confidence interval for kappa is thus $0.780 - 1.96 \times 0.0692$ to $0.780 + 1.96 \times 0.0692$, that is from 0.64 to 0.92.

The calculation of kappa can be extended quite easily to assessments with more than two categories.[2] If there are g categories and f_i is the number of agreements for the ith category, then the overall observed agreement is

$$p_o = \left(\sum_{i=1}^{g} f_i \right) \bigg/ n.$$

If r_i and c_i are the totals of the ith row and ith column, then the overall expected agreement is

$$p_e = \left(\sum_{i=1}^{g} r_i c_i \right) \bigg/ n^2.$$

Kappa and its standard error are then calculated as before.

Kappa can also be extended to multiple observers, and it is possible to weight the disagreements according to the number of categories separating the two assessments.

1 Harper R, Reeves B. Reporting of precision of estimates for diagnostic accuracy: a review. *BMJ* 1999;**318**:1322–3.
2 Altman DG. *Practical statistics for medical research*. London: Chapman & Hall, 1991:403–19.
3 Reid MC, Lachs MS, Feinstein AR. Use of methodological standards in diagnostic test research. *JAMA* 1995;**274**:645–51.
4 Deeks JJ, Altman DG. Sensitivity and specificity and their confidence intervals cannot exceed 100%. *BMJ* 1999;**318**:193–4.
5 Petersen T, Chandiramani V, Fowler CJ. The ice-water test in detrusor hyperreflexia and bladder instability. *Br J Urol* 1997;**79**:163–7.
6 Simel DL, Samsa GP, Matchar DB. Likelihood ratios with confidence: sample size estimation for diagnostic test studies. *J Clin Epidemiol* 1991;**44**:763–70.
7 Gart JJ, Nam J. Approximate interval estimation of the ratio of binomial proportions: a review and corrections for skewness. *Biometrics* 1988;**44**:323–38.
8 Nam J. Confidence limits for the ratio of two binomial proportions based on likelihood scores: non-iterative method. *Biom J* 1995;**37**:375–9.
9 Koopman PAR. Confidence limits of the ratio of two binomial proportions. *Biometrics* 1984;**80**:513–17.
10 Sackett DL, Richardson WS, Rosenberg W, Haynes RB. *Evidence-based medicine. How to practise and teach EBM*. London: Churchill-Livingstone, 1997:124.
11 Hanley JA, McNeil BJ. The meaning and use of the area under a receiver operating characteristic (ROC) curve. *Radiology* 1982;**143**:29–36.
12 Zweig MH, Campbell G. Receiver-operating characteristic (ROC) plots: a fundamental tool in clinical medicine. *Clin Chem* 1993;**39**:561–77.

13 Bagot M, Mary J-Y, Heslan M *et al.* The mixed epidermal cell lymphocyte reaction is the most predictive factor of acute graft-versus-host disease in bone marrow graft recipients. *Br J Haematol* 1988;**70**:403–9.

14 DeLong ER, DeLong DM, Clarke-Pearson DL. Comparing the areas under two or more correlated receiver operating characteristic curves: a nonparametric approach. *Biometrics* 1988;**44**:837–45.

15 Hanley JA, Haijan-Tilaki KO. Sampling variability of nonparametric estimates of the areas under receiver operating characteristic curves: an update. *Acad Radiol* 1997;**4**:49–58.

16 Obuchowski NA, Lieber ML. Confidence intervals for the receiver operating characteristic area in studies with small samples. *Acad Radiol* 1998;**5**:561–71.

17 Fooks J, Mutch L, Yudkin P, Johnson A, Elbourne D. Comparing two methods of follow up in a multicentre randomised trial. *Arch Dis Child* 1997;**76**:369–76.

11 Clinical trials and meta-analyses

DOUGLAS G ALTMAN

Confidence intervals are of special importance in the interpretation of the results of randomised clinical trials. The decision about whether or not to adopt a particular treatment is aided by knowledge of the uncertainty of the treatment effect. Most of the necessary statistical methods have been presented in earlier chapters. Here their relevance to controlled trials will be pointed out and confidence intervals for a few further measures introduced. The use of confidence intervals in meta-analyses of the data from several randomised trials is also considered.

I shall assume that two treatments are being compared. These are referred to as treatment and control, where the control group may receive an active treatment, no treatment, or placebo. There are some comments on the case of more than two groups in chapter 13.

The confidence interval indicates uncertainty in the estimated treatment effect arising from sampling variation. Note again that it does not take account of any additional uncertainty that might relate to other aspects such as the non-representativeness of the patients in a randomised trial or the studies in a meta-analysis.

Randomised controlled trials

I consider first trials using a parallel group design and then trials using the crossover design.

Parallel group trials

Continuous outcome

When the outcome is a continuous measure, such as blood pressure or lung function, the usual analysis is a comparison of the observed mean (or perhaps mean change from baseline) in the two treatment groups, using the method based on the t distribution (chapter 4).

Worked example

A randomised controlled trial compared intermittent cyclical etidronate with placebo in patients undergoing long-term oral corticosteroid therapy. The groups were compared with respect to percentage change in lumbar spine bone mineral density after two years.[1] The mean percentage increase in bone mineral density was 5·12% (SD 4·67%) in 21 etidronate-treated patients and 0·98% (SD 5·88%) in 16 placebo-treated patients. (Note that some "increases" were negative.) Using the method described in chapter 4, the mean difference between the two groups was 4·14% with standard error 1·733%. The value of $t_{0.975}$ with $21 + 16 - 2 = 35$ degrees of freedom is 2·030. A 95% confidence interval for the difference between the groups is thus

$$4·14 - 2·030 \times 1·733 \quad \text{to} \quad 4·14 + 2·030 \times 1·733$$

that is, 0·62% to 7·66%.

If the data within each treatment group are not close to having a Normal distribution, we may need to make a log transformation of the data before analysis (described in chapter 4) or use a non-parametric method (described in chapter 5).

Binary outcome

Many trials have outcomes that are binary, often indicating whether or not the patient experienced a particular event (such as a myocardial infarction or resolution of the illness). When the outcome is binary, there are three statistics commonly used to summarise the treatment effect—the risk difference, the relative risk, and the odds ratio. Methods for constructing confidence intervals for all of these measures were presented in chapters 6 and 7; here I recast them in the context of clinical trials. None of them is uniformly the most appropriate. However, the odds ratio is not an obvious effect measure for a randomised trial, and it may mislead when events are common (say >30% of patients).[2]

The data from a controlled trial can be presented as in Table 11.1. The observed proportions experiencing the event are $p_T = a/n_T$ and $p_C = b/n_C$ The *risk difference* (also called the *absolute risk reduction*) is given by $p_T - p_C$ or $p_C - p_T$, whichever is

Table 11.1 Patient outcome by treatment group

Event occurred	Group	
	Treatment	Control
Yes	a	b
No	c	d
Total	n_T	n_C

more appropriate. The appropriate confidence interval is that for the difference between two proportions, as given in chapter 6.

The *relative risk* (also called the *risk ratio*) (RR) is defined as the ratio of the event rates, either p_T/p_C or p_C/p_T. The *odds ratio* (OR) is defined as $p_T(1 - p_C)/p_C(1 - p_T)$; it is more easily obtained as ad/bc. Confidence intervals for both the relative risk and odds ratio were given in chapter 7 in the sections on incidence studies and unmatched case-control studies respectively.

Worked example

Rai et al.[3] carried out a randomised controlled trial of aspirin plus heparin versus aspirin in pregnant women with recurrent miscarriage. The proportions of women having a successful live birth was 32/45 (71%) in the aspirin plus heparin group and 19/45 (42%) in the aspirin-only group. The relative risk of a live birth was thus $R = (32/45)/(19/45) = 1.68$ and $\log_e R = 0.226$. Using the method in chapter 7, the standard error of the log relative risk is given by

$$\mathrm{SE}(\log_e R) = \sqrt{\frac{1}{32} - \frac{1}{45} + \frac{1}{19} - \frac{1}{45}} = 0.199.$$

The 95% confidence interval for $\log_e R$ is thus 0.132 to 0.911 and the 95% confidence interval for the relative risk is obtained as $e^{0.132}$ to $e^{0.911}$, or 1.14 to 2.49.

The term "relative risk" is more often used when the outcome is an adverse one. In this trial we could calculate the relative risk of failing to have a live birth. The relative risk is now $(13/45)/(26/45) = 0.5$, indicating a halving of the risk of an adverse outcome. A 95% confidence interval for $\log_e R$ is -1.215 to -0.171, and the 95% confidence interval for the relative risk is 0.30 to 0.84. These values cannot be obtained simply from those for the relative risk of a live birth.

Some authors present results using the odds ratio. This has the advantage that it gives a unique answer whether one takes a good or bad outcome. But, as noted above, it may be misleading when events are common as here. In their paper, Rai et al.[3] gave the odds ratio for a live birth as 3.37 (95% confidence interval 1.40 to 8.10). Because live births were common the odds ratio is much larger than the corresponding relative risk of 1·68. Interpreted (wrongly) as a relative risk it would imply an effect twice the size of the true one.

When the treatment of interest reduces the risk of an adverse event, so that the relative risk or odds ratio is less than 1, it may be useful to present the relative risk reduction or relative odds reduction, defined as $1 - RR$ or $1 - OR$, with a confidence interval. These values are sometimes multiplied by 100 to give percentages. In each case, the confidence interval is obtained by making the same manoeuvre. In the above study, the relative risk of not having a live birth was 0·50 with 95% confidence interval from 0·30 to 0·84. This translates into a relative risk reduction of 50% with 95% confidence interval from 16% to 70%.

A further way of quantifying the treatment effect from trials with a binary outcome is the number needed to treat. I discuss this concept later in this chapter.

Outcome is time to an event

In many studies with a binary outcome the focus of interest is not just whether an event occurred but also when it occurred. The methods used to analyse such data go under the general name of *survival analysis*, regardless of whether the outcome is death or something else. A better general name is thus *analysis of time to event data* (see chapter 9).

The outcome in such studies is often summarised as the median survival time in each group. The treatment effect is not usually summarised as the difference between these medians, however. It is not simple to provide a confidence interval, and medians often cannot be estimated when the event rate is low. Rather, it is more common to present the hazard ratio, estimated in one of the ways described in chapter 9.

Adjusting for other variables

In some trials there is ancillary information about patients which may influence the observed treatment effect. In particular, many trials with continuous outcomes collect baseline measurements of the variable that the treatment is intended to influence. The best approach for incorporating baseline values into the analysis is to use the baseline value as a predictor (covariate) in a multiple regression analysis,[4] as described in chapter 8. In other words, we perform a multiple regression of the final value on the treatment (as a binary indicator) and the baseline value. This analysis is sometimes called *analysis of covariance*; it was used in the etidronate study described earlier.[1] The regression coefficient and confidence interval from the multiple regression analysis give the adjusted treatment effect.

Other (possibly) prognostic variables are handled in the same way, being entered as explanatory variables in a multiple regression analysis. An example was given in Figure 8.3. This more general situation applies to all types of outcome and hence also to logistic and Cox regression models for binary and survival time outcomes respectively (see chapter 8). The choice of which variables to adjust for should ideally be specified in the study protocol, not by which variables seem to differ at baseline between the treatment groups.[5]

The number needed to treat

The valuable concept of the *number needed to treat* (NNT) was introduced by Laupacis *et al.*[6] as an additional way of assessing the treatment benefit from trials with a binary outcome. It has become popular as a useful way of reporting the results of clinical trials,[7] especially in journals of secondary publication (such as *ACP Journal Club* and *Evidence-Based Medicine*).

From the result of a randomised trial comparing a new treatment with a standard treatment, the NNT is the number of patients who need to be treated with the new treatment rather than the standard (control) treatment in order for one additional patient to benefit. It can be obtained for any trial that has reported a binary outcome.

The NNT is calculated as the reciprocal of the risk difference (absolute risk reduction, or ARR), given by $1/(p_C - p_T)$ (or $1/(p_T - p_C)$ if the outcome is beneficial to the patient). A large treatment effect thus leads to a small NNT. A treatment which will lead to one saved life per 10 patients treated is clearly better than a competing treatment that saves one life for every 50 treated. When there is no treatment effect the risk difference is zero and the NNT is infinite.

A confidence interval for the NNT is obtained simply by taking reciprocals of the values defining the confidence interval for the absolute risk reduction (see chapter 6). To take an example, if the risk difference in a trial is 10% with a 95% confidence interval from 5% to 15%, the NNT is $1/0 \cdot 1 = 10$ and the 95% confidence interval for the NNT is 6·7 to 20 (i.e. $1/0 \cdot 15$ to $1/0 \cdot 05$).

The case of a treatment effect that is not significant is more difficult. The same finding of ARR $= 10\%$ with a wider 95% confidence interval for the ARR of -5% to 25% gives the 95% confidence interval for the NNT of 10 as -20 to 4. There are two difficulties with this interval: first, the NNT can only be positive, and second the confidence interval does not seem to include the best estimate of 10. To avoid such perplexing results, the NNT is often given without a confidence interval when the treatments are not statistically significantly different. This is unsatisfactory behaviour, and goes against advice that the confidence interval is especially useful when the result of a trial is not statistically significant (chapter 14). In fact, a sensible confidence interval can be quoted for any trial.

In the example, the 95% confidence interval for the NNT was -20 to 4. The value of -20 indicates that if 20 patients are treated with the new treatment one *fewer* would have a good outcome than if they all received the standard treatment. In this case the inverse of the ARR is the number of patients treated for one to be harmed. This has been termed the *number needed to harm* (NNH).[8,9] However, it is more appropriate to indicate the number needed to treat for benefit (NNTB) or harm (NNTH). Using these descriptors, the value of -20 corresponds to a NNTH of 20. The confidence interval can thus be rewritten as NNTH 20 to NNTB 4. As already noted, this interval does not seem to include the overall estimate of NNTB 10.

The 95% confidence interval for the ARR includes all values of the ARR from -5% to $+25\%$, including zero. The NNT is infinity (∞) when the ARR is zero, so the confidence interval calculated as NNTH 20 to NNTB 4 must include infinity. The confidence interval is thus most peculiar, comprising values of NNTB from 4 to infinity and values of NNTH from 20 to infinity. Figure 11.1 shows the ARR and 95% confidence interval for the example. The values NNTB $= 1$ and NNTH $= 1$ thus correspond to impossible absolute risk reductions of $+100\%$ and -100% respectively, and are not actually shown. Conversely, the midpoint on the NNT scale is the case where the treatment makes no difference (ARR $= 0$ and NNT $= \infty$). We need to remember the absolute risk reduction scale when trying to interpret the NNT and its confidence interval.

It is desirable to give a confidence interval for the NNT even when the confidence interval for the absolute risk reduction

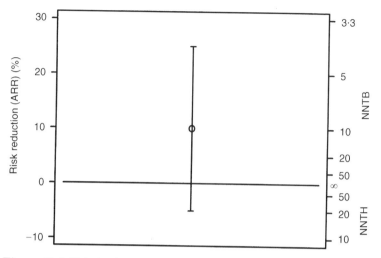

Figure 11.1 Relation between absolute risk reduction and number needed to treat and their confidence intervals for the example discussed in the text.

includes zero. I suggest that it is done as, for example, NNTB 10 (95% confidence interval NNTH 20 to ∞ to NNTB 4).

Example

Tramèr et al.[10] quoted an NNT of −12·5 for a trial comparing the antiemetic efficacy of intravenous ondansetron and intravenous droperidol. The negative NNT implies here that ondansetron was less effective than droperidol. The quoted 95% confidence interval was −3·7 to ∞, which is incomplete. The ARR was −0·08 with 95% confidence interval −0·27 to 0.11. We can convert this finding to the NNT scale as NNTH = 12.5 (95% confidence interval NNTH 3·7 to ∞ to NNTB 9·1). With this presentation we can see that an NNTB smaller (better) than 9·1 is unlikely.

The NNT can also be obtained for survival analysis. For these studies the NNT is not a single number, but varies according to time since the start of treatment.[11]

Benefit per 1000 patients

One of the arguments for using the NNT rather than the absolute risk difference is that the latter is harder to assimilate. For example, it is felt that an NNT of, say, 17 is easier to judge (and remember) than the equivalent absolute risk reduction of

5·9%. One way of representing differences between proportions that has some of the appeal of the NNT is to convert to the number of patients out of 1000 who would benefit from the new treatment. Even though this change is trivial, being achieved simply by multiplying by 10, it does simplify the results. For this measure, of course, a larger number is better.

For example, among patients randomised to streptokinase or placebo within 6 hours of their myocardial infarction, the survival rates by 35 days were 91·8% and 87·5% respectively.[12] The risk difference was thus 4·3% (95% confidence interval 2·1% to 6·5%). Baigent et al.[12] reported this result as 43 patients out of 1000 benefiting from streptokinase (95% confidence interval 21 to 65).

Crossover trials

In crossover trials patients are randomised to groups which receive each treatment in a different sequence. In the most common case, two treatments are given in one of two orders (randomly chosen for each participant), often with a "washout" period in between. The strength of the crossover design is that the two treatments are compared on the same patients rather than on two separate groups. With such trials there is no issue of comparability of groups, but there are other methodological and practical difficulties;[13] I will not dwell upon them here. Exactly the same analysis issues (and similar methodological problems) arise in within-person randomised trials.

The main difference from parallel group trials is the need to use an analysis that takes account of the paired responses for each patient in the trial. As for parallel group trials, it is essential that the confidence interval relates to the difference between treatments, not separately for the average effects with each of the treatments.

Continuous outcome

For continuous outcomes a confidence interval for the treatment effect is obtained using the method for paired continuous data presented in chapter 4.

Binary outcome

Paired binary data can be presented as in Table 11.2. As noted earlier in this chapter, the analysis of trials with binary

Table 11.2 Patient outcome (yes or no) by treatment for a clinical trial with a paired design

Control	Treatment		Total
	Yes	No	
Yes	a	b	$a + b$
No	c	d	$c + d$
Total	$a + c$	$b + d$	n

outcomes can be based on the risk difference, the relative risk, or the odds ratio. Methods for risk differences and odds ratios derived from paired binary data were presented in chapters 6 and 7 respectively.

In some crossover or within-person trials the risk difference may be felt to be the appropriate outcome measure. From Table 11.2, the proportions with a good outcome are $p_T = (a + c)/n$ and $p_C = (a + b)/n$, and thus the relative risk is estimated as $R = (a + c)/(a + b)$.

As with the unpaired case, a confidence interval can be constructed for the logarithm of the relative risk. Væth and Poulsen[14] have shown that the standard error of the log relative risk from paired data is

$$\mathrm{SE}(\log_e R) = \sqrt{\frac{1}{a + b} + \frac{1}{a + c} - \frac{2a}{(a + b)(a + c)}}.$$

The $100(1 - \alpha)\%$ confidence interval for $\log_e R$ is found by first calculating the quantities

$$W = \log_e R - z_{1 - \alpha/2} \times \mathrm{SE}(\log_e R)$$

and

$$X = \log_e R + z_{1 - \alpha/2} \times \mathrm{SE}(\log_e R).$$

As with the unpaired case (chapter 7), the confidence interval for the population relative risk is obtained by taking the antilogs of the values representing the confidence interval for $\log_e R$, namely e^W to e^X.

Worked example

Women requiring oestrogen replacement who had previously experienced skin reactions were randomly allocated to receive either a matrix

Table 11.3 Numbers of women discontinuing each type of transdermal oestradiol patch because of skin irritation[15]

Matrix	Reservoir		
	Discontinue	Continue	Total
Discontinue	9	4	13
Continue	26	33	59
Total	35	37	72

patch or a reservoir patch for eight weeks followed by the other patch for eight weeks.[15] Seventy-two women completed the study. The numbers discontinuing because of skin irritation are shown in Table 11.3.

The proportions discontinuing were 13/72 (18%) with the matrix patch and 35/72 (49%) with the reservoir patch, giving an estimated relative risk of $R = 13/35 = 0.371$. The log relative risk is $\log_e R = -0.9904$. Using the above formula, the standard error of $\log_e R$ is

$$\text{SE}(\log_e R) = \sqrt{\frac{1}{13} + \frac{1}{35} - \frac{2 \times 9}{13 \times 35}} = 0.2568.$$

The 95% confidence interval for $\log_e R$ is $\log_e R - 1.96 \times 0.2568$ to $\log_e R + 1.96 \times 0.2568$, or -1.49 to -0.487. The 95% confidence interval for the relative risk R is thus $e^{-1.49}$ to $e^{-0.487}$, or 0.22 to 0.61.

Multiple groups

Some trials have more than two treatment groups. Confidence intervals can be constructed using the methods given above for any pair of groups. The question of whether to make any allowance for multiple testing is considered in chapter 13.

Subgroups

Comparing P values alone can be misleading. Comparing confidence intervals is less likely to mislead. However, the best approach here is to compare directly the sizes of the treatment effects.[16] When comparing two independent estimates with standard errors (SE_1 and SE_2) we can derive the standard error of the difference very simply as $\text{SE}_{\text{diff}} = \sqrt{\text{SE}_1^2 + \text{SE}_2^2}$. Much the same procedure for comparing subgroups applies to all outcome measures, although the details may vary. (For continuous data we might prefer to use the method based on pooling the standard deviations, as described in chapter 4.

Table 11.4 Serum calcium levels at one week (mmol/l)

Serum calcium	Breast fed		Bottle fed	
	Supplement	Placebo	Supplement	Placebo
Treatment mean	2·45	2·41	2·30	2·20
Standard error	0·036	0·032	0·022	0·019
n	64	102	169	285
Treatment effect		0·04		0·10
Standard error		0·048		0·029
P		0·40		0·0006

It will give very similar answers unless the two standard deviations differ considerably.) A confidence interval can be constructed in the usual way (as described in chapters 4 and 6), using the difference in estimates $\pm z_{1-\alpha/2} \text{SE}_{\text{diff}}$ or $\pm t_{1-\alpha/2} \text{SE}_{\text{diff}}$ as appropriate.

Worked example

In a study of the effect of vitamin D supplementation for the prevention of neonatal hypocalcaemia[17] expectant mothers were given either supplements or placebo and the serum calcium of the baby was measured at one week. The benefit of supplementation was reported separately for breast- and bottle-fed infants, and t tests to compare the treatment groups gave P = 0·40 in the breast fed group and P = 0·0006 in the bottle-fed group (Table 11.4). It is wrong to infer that vitamin D supplementation had a different effect on breast- and bottle-fed babies on the basis of these two P values.

The estimated effect of vitamin D supplementation was 0·04 mmol/l (95% confidence interval −0·07 to +0·15 mmol/l) in 166 breast-fed babies and 0·10 mmol/l (95% confidence interval +0·04 to +0·16 mmol/l) in 454 bottle-fed babies.[16] The 95% confidence intervals for the two groups thus overlap considerably.

The difference in treatment effects in the two subgroups was $0·10 - 0·04 = 0·06$ mmol/l. Using the preceding method, the standard error of this difference is obtained as $\sqrt{0·048^2 + 0·029^2} = 0·0561$. Because of the large sample size we can use the Normal approximation to the t distribution to calculate a confidence interval. (If we use the t method there are $N - 4$ degrees of freedom for the t statistic where N is the total trial size.)

The 95% confidence interval for the contrast between the groups is thus $0·06 - 1·96 \times 0·0561$ to $0·06 + 1·96 \times 0·0561$, or −0·05 to 0·17 mmol/l. There is thus no good evidence that the effect of vitamin D supplementation differs between breast- and bottle-fed infants.

Table 11.5 Outcomes after intensive insulin treatment versus standard treatment following myocardial infarction[21]

Outcomes	Intensive insulin event rate	Standard treatment event rate	Relative risk reduction (95% CI)	Absolute risk reduction (95% CI)	NNT (95% CI)
Death at 1 year	19%	26%	27% (2·5 to 46)	7%	15 (7 to 172)
Death at mean of 3·4 years	33%	44%	24% (7·3 to 38)	11%	10 (6 to 34)

Presentation

There are few problems regarding the presentation of confidence intervals from clinical trials, other than for the NNT as discussed already. One point worth emphasising is that the confidence interval should always be presented for the difference in outcome between the treatment groups. It is a common error to present instead separate confidence intervals for the means or event rates observed in each group. A similar error is to calculate the confidence interval associated with change from baseline in each group. This error has been noted in about 10% of published trials.[18,19]

Confidence intervals are widely used in journals of secondary publication, in which each study is given one journal page which includes both a summary of the paper and a short commentary on it. An example of the style of presentation is given Table 11.5, which summarises the results of a randomised trial comparing intensive versus standard insulin treatment after acute myocardial infarction in diabetics[20] as presented in *Evidence-Based Medicine*.

In recent years many journals have begun to require authors to present confidence intervals in their papers, especially for the principal outcomes. Particular attention has been given to randomised controlled trials, culminating in the CONSORT statement.[22] These guidelines, which have been adopted by over 70 journals, include the requirement that authors present confidence intervals. Reporting of results is considered in more depth in chapters 14 and 15.

Interpretation

The interpretation of confidence intervals has been discussed earlier, notably in chapter 3. There should be no special problems relating to trials. Confidence intervals are especially useful in

131

association with trials which have not found a significant treatment benefit, as they indicate a range of possible true effects with which the results are compatible. Given that many trials are too small to have adequate power to detect modest yet clinically valuable benefits,[23] the width of the confidence interval can signal the danger of interpreting "no significant difference" as "no difference". Sadly, authors sometimes ignore the confidence interval when interpreting their results. For example, Sung *et al.*[24] randomised patients to octreotide infusion or emergency sclerotherapy for acute variceal haemorrhage. They randomised 100 patients despite a power calculation showing that they needed 1800 patients to have reasonable power to detect an improvement in response rate from 85% to 90%. The observed rates of controlled bleeding were 84% in the octreotide group and 90% in the sclerotherapy group. They quoted a confidence interval for the treatment difference as 0 to 19%—it should have been −7% to 19%. More seriously, they drew the unjustified conclusion that "octreotide infusion and sclerotherapy are equally effective in controlling variceal haemorrhage".

Meta-analysis

Many systematic reviews of the literature include a statistical meta-analysis to combine the results of several similar studies. There is a clear need to present confidence intervals when summarising a body of literature. This section considers meta-analyses of randomised trials. Much the same considerations apply to meta-analyses of other types of study, including epidemiological studies.

I will not describe here methods of performing meta-analysis, but will focus instead on the use of confidence intervals in the display of results.

Analysis

Meta-analysis is a two-stage analysis. For each trial a summary of the treatment effect is calculated and then a weighted average of these estimates is obtained, where the weights relate to the precision of each study's estimate (effectively, the width of the confidence interval). There are various methods of meta-analysis for both binary and continuous data.[25,26] In each case, a confidence interval is obtained from the pooled estimate and its standard error using the general formula given in chapter 3. Confidence intervals feature prominently in the presensation of results of meta-analyses.

For any type of outcome an analysis may used a "fixed" or "random" effects approach. The former considers only the data to hand whereas the latter assumes that the studies are representative of some larger population of trials that might have been performed.[25,26] Although in many cases the two methods agree quite closely, the random effects approach gives wider confidence intervals because it allows for an additional element of uncertainty.

Continuous outcome

The principal methods for performing meta-analysis of trials with continuous outcomes are the weighted mean difference and the standardised (weighted) mean difference. These methods yield a mean effect with a standard error, so confidence intervals are easily calculated using the general approach outlined in chapter 3.

Binary outcome

As for single trials, meta-analysis of several similar trials with a binary outcome can be based on the risk difference, the relative risk, or the odds ratio. None can be considered to be the best for all circumstances. The Mantel–Haenszel method is commonly used. It was described in chapter 7 in the context of stratified case-control studies. Although most familiar as a means of combining odds ratios, there are also versions of the Mantel–Haenszel method for obtaining either a pooled relative risk or risk difference.[27]

Worked example

Figure 11.2 shows the risk ratio associated with coronary artery bypass grafting versus coronary angioplasty and its 95% confidence interval for each trial and for the overall estimate (based on a fixed effect analysis). The four smallest trials have been combined.[28] For each trial the risk ratio and 95% confidence interval are shown both numerically and graphically. The size of the black boxes is proportional to the weight given to each trial's results in the meta-analysis. The diamond represents the overall treatment effect (also shown by the dashed line) and its 95% confidence interval, obtained by combining the results of the eight trials.

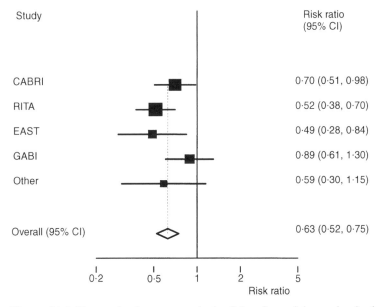

Figure 11.2 Forest plot for meta-analysis of data from eight randomised trials relating to angina in one year comparing coronary artery bypass surgery with coronary angioplasty.[28]

Outcome is time to an event

Meta-analysis of trials is also possible where the outcome is time to an event. There are serious practical problems, however, as many published papers do not provide the necessary information. Acquiring the raw data from all studies, while desirable, is rarely feasible. Some methods based on published summary statistics have been described by Parmar *et al.*[29]

Presentation

Although tables are helpful in meta-analyses, especially to show the actual summary data from each trial, it is usual to show graphically the results of all the trials with their confidence intervals. The most common type of plot is called a *forest plot*. Such plots tabulate the summary results, estimates and confidence intervals for each study, and depict these graphically. Sometimes the weight given to each trial is also shown. A simplified example is shown in Figure 11.2.

When the effect size has been summarised as relative risk or odds ratio the analysis is based on the logarithms of these values. The

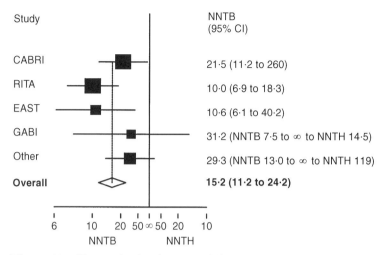

Figure 11.3 Forest plot for the same trials as shown in fig 11.2, showing NNTB for coronary artery bypass surgery and its 95% confidence interval for each trial and for the overall estimate. The four smallest trials have been combined.

forest plot benefits from using a log scale for the treatment effect as the confidence intervals for each trial are then symmetric around the estimate (see Figure 11.2).

It is common to use 95% confidence intervals both for each trial and for the overall pooled effect, but some authors use wider confidence intervals (often 99%) for the pooled estimate on the grounds that one is looking for convincing evidence regarding treatment benefit, while others use 99% confidence intervals for the results of each trial.

A forest plot can also be made using the NNT. Noting, as before, that the NNT should be plotted on the absolute risk reduction scale, it is relatively simple to plot NNTs with confidence intervals for multiple trials, even when (as is usual) some of the trials did not show statistically significant results. Figure 11.3 shows such a plot for the same trials as in Figure 11.2. The plot was produced using the absolute risk reduction scale, and then relabelled (this cannot be done in many software packages). Both scales can be shown in the figure.

Interpretation

As already noted, confidence intervals are an especially important feature of meta-analyses. Systematic reviews of the literature aim to provide a reliable answer based on all available evidence. It is important to know not just the average overall effect but also to be able to see how much uncertainty is associated with that estimate.

Software

CIA can perform all of the methods described for randomised controlled trials, but not those for meta-analysis, for which specialist software is advisable.

Comment

I have shown how the analysis of clinical trials, including the calculation of confidence intervals, varies for parallel and crossover trials, corresponding to whether the data are unpaired or paired respectively. Some other trial designs also affect the analysis. This applies in particular to cluster randomised trials, in which patients are randomised in groups, such as those with a particular general practitioner or attending a particular hospital. For such trials analysis of individual patient data is misleading and will lead to confidence intervals which are too narrow. It is essential that the analysis of such trials is based on the randomised clusters.[30]

Although the focus of interest in this chapter has been on primary treatment effects, there is a similar need to provide confidence intervals for other outcomes, including adverse events and cost data. Such information is usually missing from published reports.[31]

1 Pitt P, Li F, Todd P, Webber D, Pack S, Moniz C. A double blind placebo controlled study to determine the effects of intermittent cyclical etidronate on bone mineral density in patients undergoing long term oral corticosteroid therapy. *Thorax* 1998;**53**:351–6.

2 Sackett DL, Deeks JJ, Altman DG. Down with odds ratios! *Evidence-Based Med* 1996;**1**:164–6.

3 Rai R, Cohen H, Dave M, Regan L. Randomised controlled trial of aspirin and aspirin plus heparin in pregnant women with recurrent miscarriage associated with phospholipid antibodies (or antiphospholipid antibodies). *BMJ* 1997; **314**:253–7.

4 Senn S. Baselines and covariate information. In: *Statistical issues in drug development*. Chichester: John Wiley, 1997:95–109.

5 Altman DG. Covariate imbalance, adjustment for. In: Armitage P, Colton T (eds) *Encyclopedia of biostatistics*. Chichester: John Wiley, 1998: 1000–5.

6 Laupacis A, Sackett DL, Roberts RS. An assessment of clinically useful measures of the consequences of treatment. *N Engl J Med* 1988;**318**:1728–33.

7 Cook RJ, Sackett DL. The number needed to treat: a clinically useful measure of treatment effect. *BMJ* 1995;**310**:452–4.

8 McQuay HJ, Moore RA. Using numerical results from systematic reviews in clinical practice. *Ann Intern Med* 1997;**126**:712–20.

9 Sackett DL, Richardson WS, Rosenberg W, Haynes RB. *Evidence-based medicine. How to practise and teach EBM*. London: Churchill-Livingstone, 1997: 208.

10 Tramèr MR, Moore, RA, Reynolds DJM, McQuay HJ. A quantitative systematic review of ondansetron in treatment of established postoperative nausea and vomiting. *BMJ* 1997;**314**:1088–92.

11 Altman DG, Andersen PK. Calculating the number needed to treat for trials where the outcome is time to an event. *BMJ* 1999; **319**:1492–5.

12 Baigent C, Collins R, Appleby P, Parish S, Sleight P, Peto R. ISIS-2: 10 year survival among patients with suspected acute myocardial infarction in randomised comparison of intravenous streptokinase, oral aspirin, both, or neither. *BMJ* 1998;**316**:1337–43.

13 Senn S. *Cross-over trials in clinical research*. Chichester: John Wiley, 1993.

14 Væth M, Poulsen S. Comments on a commentary: statistical evaluation of split mouth caries trials. *Community Dent Oral Epidemiol* 1998;**26**:80–3.

15 Ross D, Rees M, Godfree V, Cooper A, Hart D, Kingland C, Whitehead M. Randomised crossover comparison of skin irritation with two transdermal oestradiol patches. *BMJ* 1997;**317**:288.

16 Matthews JNS, Altman DG. Interaction 3: How to examine heterogeneity. *BMJ* 1996;**313**:862.

17 Cockbum F, Belton NR, Purvis RJ, Giles MM, *et al*. Maternal vitamin D intake and mineral metabolism in mothers and their newborn infants. *BMJ* 1980;**281**:11–14.

18 Altman DG, Doré CJ. Randomisation and baseline comparisons in clinical trials. *Lancet* 1990;**335**:149–53.

19 Gøtzsche PC. Methodology and overt and hidden bias in reports of 196 double-blind trials of non-steroidal antiinflammatory drugs in rheumatoid arthritis. *Controlled Clin Trials* 1989;**10**:31–56.

20 Malmberg K for the DIGAMI Study Group. Prospective randomised study of intensive insulin treatment on long term survival after acute myocardial infarction in patients with diabetes mellitus. *BMJ* 1997;**314**:1512–15.

21 Malmberg K for the DIGAMI Study Group. Intensive insulin regimen reduced long-term mortality after MI in diabetes mellitus. *Evidence-Based Med* 1997;**2**:173.

22 Begg C, Cho M, Eastwood S, Horton R, Moher D, Olkin I, *et al*. Improving the quality of reporting of randomized controlled trials: the CONSORT statement. *JAMA* 1996;**276**:637–9.

23 Thornley B, Adams C. Content and quality of 2000 controlled trials in schizophrenia over 50 years. *BMJ* 1998;**317**:1181–4.

24 Sung JJY, Chung SCS, Lai C-W, Chan FKL, *et al*. Octreotide infusion or emergency sclerotherapy for variceal haemorrhage. *Lancet* 1993;**342**:637–41.

25 Fleiss JL. The statistical basis of meta-analysis. *Stat Meth Med Res* 1993;**2**:121–45.

26 DerSimonian R, Laird N. Meta-analysis in clinical trials. *Controlled Clin Trials* 1986;**7**:177–86.

27 Greenland S, Robins J. Estimation of a common effect parameter from sparse follow-up data. *Biometrics* 1985;**41**;55–68.

28 Pocock SJ, Henderson RA, Rickards AF, Hampton JR, King SB, Hamm CW *et al*. Meta-analysis of randomised trials comparing coronary angioplasty with bypass surgery. *Lancet* 1995;**346**:1184–9.

29 Parmar M, Torri V, Stewart L. Extracting summary statistics to perform meta-analyses of the published literature for survival endpoints. *Stat Med* 1998;**117**:2815–34.

30 Kerry SM, Bland JM. Analysis of a trial randomised in clusters. *BMJ* 1998;**316**:54.

31 Barber JA, Thompson SG. Analysis and interpretation of cost data in randomised controlled trials: review of published studies. *BMJ* 1998;**317**:1195–200.

12 Confidence intervals and sample sizes

LESLIE E DALY

A major part of the planning of any investigation is the estimation of an appropriate sample size. In line with the move towards confidence intervals in data analysis, a number of sample size estimation methods based on that philosophy have been proposed as alternatives to the more traditional methods based on hypothesis testing. These newer methods just require a pre-specification of a target confidence interval width and are much easier to understand.

If the sole purpose of an investigation is to obtain an estimate for a non-comparative measure (for example, in a descriptive prevalence study where no comparisons are planned) then sample size calculations based on confidence interval width are perfectly acceptable. In this chapter, however I argue that for comparative studies, the confidence interval width approach, though appearing to have many advantages, leads to unacceptably small sample sizes. For such studies the traditional sample size formulae should always be employed. These formulae can, however, be made fully compatible with a confidence interval approach to data analysis with an appropriate change in the wording and interpretation of the specification.

The discussion is illustrated using the comparison of both means and percentages in two independent equal-sized groups using difference measures. The arguments, however, extend to unequal sample sizes, to the use of other measures (for example, ratios of means or relative risks) and to within-subjects designs such as crossover trials.

Confidence intervals and P values

A large proportion of medical research involves the comparison of two groups, each of which may be considered a sample from a larger population in which we are interested. The hypothesis testing approach to statistical analysis determines if some appropriate comparative measure (such as a difference between means or percentages or a relative risk) is significantly different from its null value (for example a mean difference of zero or a relative risk of unity). The confidence interval approach, however, concentrates on an estimate of the comparative measure together with its confidence limits. The confidence interval gives an indication of the degree of imprecision of the sample value as an estimate of the population value. It is important to note that hypothesis testing and confidence intervals are intimately connected. If a 95% confidence interval does not include the null value of the hypothesis test then we can infer a statistically significant result at the two-sided 5% level. If the null value of the comparative measure lies inside the confidence interval then the result is not statistically significant (see chapter 3).

Sample size and hypothesis tests

Suppose we are planning a randomised controlled trial to compare an antihypertensive agent with a placebo and that suitable hypertensive patients are to be randomised into two equal-sized groups. We take two cases. The first is where the treatment effect is to be evaluated by examining the difference in mean systolic blood pressure between the groups after a period of, say, six weeks. As an alternative endpoint, to illustrate the comparison of percentages, we also take the case where the treatment effect is evaluated by examining the difference in the percentage of patients in each group who have severe hypertension (say a systolic pressure above 180 mmHg).

To determine the sample size required for such a two group comparison several quantities must be considered:[1,2]

- The *significance level* (usually 5% or 1 %) at which we wish to perform our hypothesis test, and if it is to be one sided or two sided. (Apart from exceptional circumstances two-sided tests are usually more appropriate.)
- The *smallest clinically worthwhile difference* we wish to detect. Taking the difference in mean blood pressures to illustrate what we mean, we must distinguish between the blood pressure difference that we might observe in our study (the sample result) and the real treatment effect. The real treatment

effect can be thought of as the difference in blood pressures that would be observed in a study so large that sample variation was precluded, or alternatively, as the blood pressure difference between the "populations" of treated and untreated patients. If there were a real treatment effect (that is, if the null hypothesis were false) we would want our study to reflect this and reject the null hypothesis with a statistically significant result. We would be unlikely, however, to be interested in detecting a very small (real population) difference of say only 1 mmHg since, from a clinical point of view, such a treatment effect could be considered negligible. We therefore decide on the smallest difference worth detecting such that, if the real difference was this large or larger, we would be likely to achieve a statistically significant result; on the other hand, for real differences smaller than this, a non-significant result is judged acceptable.[3] In our trial this smallest worthwhile difference might be set at 5 mmHg.

If the trial endpoint had been expressed in terms of the percentage of patients with severe hypertension rather than in terms of a mean blood pressure, the smallest difference worth detecting would be expressed as a percentage. Thus we might be interested in detecting, as statistically significant, a treatment effect that reduced the percentage with severe hypertension by 10% or more, but would accept a non-significant result if the real treatment effect were any less than this.

- The *power* of the study. This is the chance of obtaining a significant result if the real effect is as great as or greater than the smallest worthwhile difference specified. Powers of 80% or 90% are typical choices.

- For comparing means, the *variability of the measure* in the study population. This is usually determined from a pilot investigation or from published results. (Note that the approach described below assumes that the distribution of the measure is approximately Normal or at least not too skew.) For illustrative purposes we shall take the standard deviation of systolic blood pressure in hypertensives to be 20 mmHg.

- For comparing percentages, the *percentage in one of the groups*. In our example we would have to specify the percentage with severe hypertension in one of the groups instead of the standard deviation required when comparing means. We assume

Table 12.1 Sample size in each group for an independent two-group comparison of mean blood pressures, pre-specifying power to detect a smallest worthwhile difference (at a two-sided significance level of 5%). The population standard deviation is 20 mmHg

Smallest difference to be detected	Power		
	90%	80%	50%
5 mmHg	336	251	123
10 mmHg	84	63	31
15 mmHg	38	28	14

here that the percentage of controls with severe hypertension is 50%. Thus a smallest worthwhile difference of 10% would correspond to a percentage with severe hypertension of 40% in the treatment group.

Given levels for the significance, power and smallest difference (of means or percentages) to be detected and, as appropriate, a standard deviation or a percentage in controls, standard formulae, tables and graphs are available to enable calculation of the required sample size. These are reviewed by Lachin.[2] To illustrate the method, Table 12.1 gives required sample sizes, in each group of our clinical trial, for three different levels of the smallest worthwhile difference in mean blood pressure to be detected (5, 10, and 15 mmHg), and powers of 50%, 80%, and 90%. A two-sided 5% significance level, and a population blood pressure standard deviation of 20 mmHg are assumed. The required sample size increases with the power, but decreases for higher levels of the difference to be detected. For the same levels of power and significance, Table 12.2 gives sample sizes for detecting

Table 12.2 Sample size in each group for an independent two-group comparison of the percentage with severe hypertension, pre-specifying power to detect a smallest worthwhile difference (at a two-sided significance level of 5%). The percentage with severe hypertension in the controls is 50%

Smallest difference to be detected	Power		
	90%	80%	50%
10%	515	383	189
20%	121	90	45
25%	74	55	27

differences in the percentage with severe hypertension of 10%, 20% and 25% from a control level of 50%. The appendix gives the equations from which these figures are calculated.

Sample size and confidence intervals

Most of the confidence interval approaches to sample size estimation are based on the expected width of the confidence interval for the comparative measure (difference between means or percentages) being analysed. (The width of a confidence interval is a measure of the imprecision of the sample estimate and is the difference between the upper and lower confidence limits. For example, if a confidence interval were determined to be from 90 to 170, its width would be 80.) All else being equal, the larger the sample size the narrower the width of the confidence interval. Once the width has been pre-specified, the only additional requirements for a sample size determination using this approach are the confidence level (95% or 99%) and an estimate of the variability of the means or an estimate of the percentages in the groups. These specifications are clinically understandable and the difficult concepts of power, the null value and a smallest difference to be detected seem to be avoided altogether. In addition, concentration on the precision of the estimate seems to fit in fully with an analysis that is to be performed using confidence intervals. Tables and formulae using this approach are available for various comparative measures in journals[4-7] and textbooks.[8] (A further refinement is to estimate sample sizes on the basis that the width of the confidence interval, rather than being fixed, is a percentage of the actual population value.[4,5,9]) Some simple formulae for sample size determination based on confidence interval width are given in the appendix.

Confidence intervals and null values

Although the specifications of confidence level and confidence interval width for a sample size calculation are easy to understand, estimates of sample size based on this approach can be misleading. The consequences of employing such estimates do not seem to be clearly understood and in general the published work does not consider the problems explicitly. One distinction between hypothesis tests and confidence intervals is important in this regard.[10,11] Hypothesis tests are essentially asymmetrical. Emphasis is on rejection or non-rejection of the null hypothesis based on how far the observed comparative measure (in our example, the difference between means or percentages) is from the value specified by the null hypothesis (a zero difference). On the other hand, confidence intervals are symmetrical and estimate the magnitude of the difference between two groups without giving any special importance to the null value of the former approach. It seems mistaken, however, to conclude that this null value is irrelevant to the *interpretation* of confidence intervals even though it plays no part in their calculation. Irrespective of precision, there is a qualitative difference between a confidence interval which includes the null value and one which does not include it. In the former case, at the given confidence level, the possibility of no difference must be accepted, while in the latter situation some difference has been demonstrated at a given level of probability. Herein lies the crux of the problem. In a comparative study can we ever say that the primary goal is just estimation and ignore completely the qualitative distinction between a "difference" and "no difference", or in hypothesis testing terms, between a significant and a non-significant result? The answer is clearly "no" and I argue that the null value must have a central role in the estimation of sample sizes—even with a confidence interval approach—and that the position of the confidence interval is as relevant as its actual width.

Confidence intervals, power and worthwhile differences

The role of the smallest clinically worthwhile difference to be detected (as specified by the alternative hypothesis) has also been questioned in the context of sample sizes based on confidence intervals. Beal states: "With estimation as the primary goal, where construction of a confidence interval is the appropriate inferential procedure, the concept of an alternative hypothesis is inconsistent with the associated philosophy, even when used as an indirect approach to hypothesis testing. Thus one should not, in this situation, determine sample size by controlling the power at an appropriate alternative."[12] This viewpoint is untenable. For a sample size determination it seems inappropriate to specify the precision of an estimate without any consideration of what the real differences between the groups might be. Unfortunately, though the problem has been recognised by some,[10,13] others make a correspondence between the precision of the confidence

Table 12.3 Sample size in each group for an independent two-group comparison of mean blood pressures, pre-specifying confidence interval width (95% confidence interval). The population standard deviation is 20 mmHg

Confidence interval width	Sample size required
5 mmHg	123
10 mmHg	31
15 mmHg	14

interval and the smallest difference to be detected. In the clinical trial example, we might decide that a confidence interval width for blood pressure difference of just under 10 mmHg would be sufficient to distinguish a mean difference of 5 mmHg from that of a zero difference. If the confidence interval were centred around the observed difference, the expected interval of 5 ± 5 mmHg (that is, from 0 to 10 mmHg) would just exclude the null value. Similarly a confidence interval width of 20% for a difference between percentages should allow detection of a 10% difference.

Tables 12.3 and 12.4 give the sample size requirements in each group of our clinical trial to achieve confidence interval widths of 10, 20, or 30 mmHg for the difference in mean blood pressures between the groups, and to achieve confidence interval widths of 20%, 40%, and 50% for the difference in the percentage with severe hypertension. A comparison with the sample sizes based on the hypothesis test approach given in Tables 12.1 and 12.2 shows that those based on confidence intervals would have only 50% power to detect the corresponding smallest worthwhile

Table 12.4 Sample size in each group for an independent two-group comparison of the percentage with severe hypertension, pre-specifying confidence interval width (95% confidence interval). The table assumes that the width is equal to twice the difference between the population percentages, one of which is specified at 50%. See appendix

Confidence interval width	Sample size required
20%	189
40%	45
50%	27

differences. Thus even if the real difference were as large as postulated, with the confidence interval-based sample sizes there would be a 50% chance of the confidence interval overlapping zero. This would mean a statistically non-significant result and a consequent acceptance of the possibility of there being no real difference.

Explanation of the anomaly

There are two reasons for this apparent anomaly. Take the comparison of means and assume the real population blood pressure difference was in fact 5 mmHg and that, based on a pre-specified confidence interval width of 10 mmHg, a sample size of 123 was used in each group. Firstly, this width is only an expected or average width. The width we might obtain on any actual data from the study would be above its expected value about 50% of the time. Thus, the confidence interval, if centred around 5 mmHg, would have a 50% chance of including zero. Secondly, the sample value of the blood pressure difference calculated on the study results would be as likely to be above the population value of 5 mmHg as below it. If our sample estimate were, for instance, 4 mmHg, then a confidence interval, with the expected width of 10 mmHg, would run from −1 mmHg to +9 mmHg and would include zero difference as a possible true value. Thus specification of the expected width of a confidence interval as described above does not consider the possible true values of the difference and the power of detecting them (with a confidence interval excluding the null value of zero); nor does it consider what confidence interval width might actually be achieved. Consequently the approach leads to unacceptably small sample sizes with too low a power (only 50%) to detect the required effect.

Proposed solutions

Beal and Grieve propose sample size estimations based on a confidence interval width specification together with a probability (somewhat akin to power) that the width be less than a given value.[12,14–16] This overcomes the problem related to expected width discussed above but does not account for the true location of the parameter of interest. Sample sizes based on this approach are still much lower than traditional estimates.

In planning any investigation, the question of power to detect the smallest clinically worthwhile difference must predominate over that of precision. In practice, of course, estimates based on samples large enough to detect small differences will have a high degree of precision. It is only when we are trying to detect large differences (not often found in medical research) that an imprecise estimate will result. In this latter situation it would in any case be possible to calculate a sample size based on precision also and use the larger of the two sizes so calculated. In line with this view, Bristol[11] gives tables and formulae relating the width of the interval to the power for detecting various alternatives when comparing differences of means and proportions. However, if these factors have to be considered at all, why should sample size estimates not explicitly specify power to detect the smallest worthwhile difference in the first place, rather than concealing the specification in a vaguer requirement for confidence interval precision?

Confidence intervals and standard sample size tables

I propose that sample size requirements, which explicitly consider power, null values and smallest worthwhile differences, can easily be put into a confidence interval framework without the consideration of hypothesis tests in either design or analysis. Although the discussion has been in the context of employing the difference between means or percentages as a comparative measure, this proposal has general applicability. For calculation of a sample size based on a confidence interval approach we should specify (1) the confidence level (usually 95% or 99%), (2) the minimum size of the comparative measure we wish to estimate unambiguously (that is with the confidence interval excluding the null value), and (3) the chance of achieving this if the measure actually had this minimum value (in the population). These correspond, of course, to the traditional requirements of (1) the significance level, (2) the smallest worthwhile difference to be detected, and (3) the power of the study. Thus with only a slight change of wording the standard procedures based on hypothesis testing can be used to estimate sample sizes in the context of a confidence interval analysis.

In our example, we might have specified that the trial should be big enough to have an 80% chance that, if the real difference in blood pressure were 5 mmHg or greater, the 95% confidence interval for the mean difference would exclude zero. This would result in a sample size requirement of 251 in each group (see Table 12.1).

It is essential to note that this approach allows for the sampling variability of both the location and width of the confidence interval. The width of the interval, however, is not explicitly pre-specified. It is instead determined by the more important criterion that we are unlikely to miss a difference we wish to detect.

Greenland comes nearest to this view in terms of confidence intervals and sample size.[10] The proposal outlined in this chapter is based on distinguishing between a particular difference, if it exists, and the null value. Greenland, however, in a subtle modification of this approach, also suggests that the sample size be large enough to distinguish between the null value and this difference, if the groups are in fact the same. In most situations this extra requirement does not result in an increase of sample size and it seems an unnecessary refinement.

Conclusion

There is no doubt that the whole topic of traditional sample size calculation tends to be complex and misunderstood and many studies are carried out with inadequate numbers.[17,18] Estimating an appropriate sample size is a vital part of any research design and it is important that the current emphasis on using confidence intervals in analysis and presentation does not mislead researchers to employ sample sizes based on confidence interval width. Though apparently much simpler, such calculations can result in studies so small that they are unlikely to detect the very effects they are being designed to look for.

Examination of precision may well be a useful adjunct to the traditional estimation of sample size,[13] but unless we place our primary emphasis on the question of power to detect an appropriate effect, we could be making a serious mistake. The use of confidence intervals in analysis, however, must be encouraged and this chapter has indicated how a realistic rewording of the usual specifications allows standard approaches to be used for sample size calculations in a confidence interval framework.

There is no need to throw out our old sample size tables in this era of confidence intervals. In fact we should guard them with care. Inadequate sample size has been a major problem in medical research in the past and we do not want to repeat those mistakes in the future. "However praiseworthy a study may be from other points of view, if the statistical aspects are substandard then the research will be unethical."[19] If we depart from the tried and tested approach for sample size calculations we are in danger of disregarding this principle.

Appendix

Notation

This Appendix gives the formulae on which the sample size calculations in this chapter are based. Though percentages are used in the text the formulae given here, as in the rest of this book, are in terms of proportions. Significance, confidence and power levels are also expressed as proportions. All relevant quantities should be converted from percentages to proportions by dividing by 100 prior to using the formulae.

The following notation is employed:

n	Sample size in each of the two groups (the value for n given by the formulae should be rounded up to the next highest integer)
σ	Population standard deviation (assumed equal in the two groups)
μ_1, μ_2	Population means in each group
π_1, π_2	Population proportions in each group
Δ	Smallest worthwhile difference to be detected ($\mu_1 - \mu_2$ or $\pi_1 - \pi_2$)
α	Two-sided significance level
$1 - \alpha$	Confidence level
$1 - \beta$	Power of test to detect the smallest worthwhile difference Δ
z_k	$100k$th percentile of Normal distribution

Values of z_k for values of k commonly used in sample size calculations are shown below:

k	0·975	0·90	0·80	0·50
z_k	1·96	1·28	0·84	0·00

Sample size for comparison of two independent means

The sample size per group, given a specification for significance, power and the smallest difference to be detected, is

$$n = \frac{2 \times (z_{1-\alpha/2} + z_{1-\beta})^2 \times \sigma^2}{\Delta^2}$$

The expected $100(1 - \alpha)\%$ confidence interval for the difference between means (using the Normal approximation) is

$$(\mu_1 - \mu_2) \pm z_{1-\alpha/2} \times \sqrt{2\sigma^2/n}.$$

(Note that the actual confidence interval for a given set of study data would use the sample means rather than the population means, the pooled estimate of the sample standard deviation rather than σ, and the appropriate critical value of the Student's t distribution rather than $z_{1-\alpha/2}$—see chapter 4.)

The expected width of the confidence interval, W, is thus

$$W = 2 \times z_{1-\alpha/2} \times \sqrt{2\sigma^2/n}.$$

Rearranging this equation, the sample size per group, based on confidence interval width, is obtained as

$$n = \frac{8 \times (z_{1-\alpha/2} \times \sigma)^2}{W^2}$$

which, if W is set equal to 2Δ, reduces to

$$n = \frac{2 \times (z_{1-\alpha/2} \times \sigma)^2}{\Delta^2}$$

Sample size based on confidence interval width is thus equal to the conventional calculation when $z_{1-\beta} = 0$, implying that $\beta = 0 \cdot 5$ and the power is 50%.

Sample size for comparison of two independent proportions

The sample size per group, given a specification for significance, power and the smallest difference to be detected, is

$$n = \frac{(z_{1-\alpha/2} + z_{1-\beta})^2 \times [\pi_1(1 - \pi_1) + \pi_2(1 - \pi_2)]}{\Delta^2}.$$

The expected $100(1 - \alpha)\%$ confidence interval for a difference between proportions (using the traditional method of chapter 6) is

$$(\pi_1 - \pi_2) \pm z_{1-\alpha/2} \times \sqrt{[\pi_1(1 - \pi_1) + \pi_2(1 - \pi_2)]/n}.$$

(Note that the actual confidence interval for a given set of study data would use the sample proportions rather than the population values. Also, chapter 6 presents more accurate formulae.)

The expected width of the confidence interval, W, is thus

$$W = 2 \times z_{1-\alpha/2} \times \sqrt{[\pi_1(1-\pi_1) + \pi_2(1-\pi_2)]/n}.$$

Rearranging this equation, the sample size per group, based on confidence interval width, is obtained as

$$n = \frac{4 \times (z_{1-\alpha/2})^2 \times [\pi_1(1-\pi_1) + \pi_2(1-\pi_2)]}{W^2}$$

which, if W is set equal to $2\Delta = 2(\pi_1 - \pi_2)$, reduces to

$$n = \frac{(z_{1-\alpha/2})^2 \times [\pi_1(1-\pi_1) + \pi_2(1-\pi_2)]}{\Delta^2}.$$

Sample size based on confidence interval width is thus equal to the conventional calculation when $z_{1-\beta} = 0$, implying that $\beta = 0.5$ and the power is 50%.

1 Donner A. Approaches to sample size estimation in the design of clinical trials – a review. *Stat Med* 1984;**3**:199-214.
2 Lachin JM. Introduction to sample size determination and power analysis for clinical trials. *Controlled Clin Trials* 1981;**2**:93–113.
3 Spiegelhalter DJ, Freedman LS. A predictive approach to selecting the size of a clinical trial, based on subjective clinical opinion. *Stat Med* 1986;**5**:1–13.
4 McHugh RB, Le CT. Confidence estimation and the size of a clinical trial. *Controlled Clin Trials* 1984;**5**:157–63.
5 O'Neill RT. Sample sizes for estimation of the odds ratio in unmatched case-control studies. *Am J Epidemiol* 1984;**120**:145–53.
6 Day SJ. Clinical trial numbers and confidence intervals of pre-specified size (Letter). *Lancet* 1988;**ii**:1427.
7 Gordon I. Sample size estimation in occupational mortality studies with use of confidence interval theory. *Am J Epidemiol* 1987;**125**:158–62.
8 Machin D, Campbell MJ, Fayers PM, Pinol APY. *Sample size tables for clinical studies*. 2nd ed. Oxford: Blackwell Science, 1997.
9 Lemeshow S, Hosmer DW, Klar J. Sample size requirements for studies estimating odds ratios or relative risks. *Stat Med* 1988;**7**:759–64.
10 Greenland S. On sample-size and power calculations for studies using confidence intervals. *Am J Epidemiol* 1988;**128**:231–7.
11 Bristol DR. Sample sizes for constructing confidence intervals and testing hypotheses. *Stat Med* 1989;**8**:803–11.
12 Beal SL. Sample size determination for confidence intervals on the population mean and on the difference between two population means. *Biometrics* 1989;**45**:969–77.
13 Goodman SN, Berlin JA. The use of predicted confidence intervals when planning experiments and the misuse of power when interpreting results. *Ann Intern Med* 1994;**121**:200–6.
14 Beal SL. Response to "Confidence intervals and sample sizes". *Biometrics* 1991;**47**:1602–3.
15 Grieve AP. Confidence intervals and trial sizes (Letter). *Lancet*. 1989;**i**:337.
16 Grieve AP. Confidence intervals and sample sizes. *Biometrics* 1991;**47**:1597–602.

17 Moher D, Dulberg CS, Wells GA. Statistical power, sample size, and their reporting in randomized controlled trials. *JAMA* 1994;**272**:122–4.
18 Thornley B, Adams C. Content and quality of 2000 controlled trials in schizophrenia over 50 years. *BMJ* 1998;**317**:1181–4.
19 Altman DG. Misuse of statistics is unethical. In: Gore SM, Altman DG. *Statistics in practice*. London: British Medical Association, 1982:1–2.

13 Special topics

MICHAEL J CAMPBELL, LESLIE E DALY,
DAVID MACHIN

In this chapter we describe some special topics relating to the construction and interpretation of confidence intervals in particular situations. Some of these methods have been referred to before in this book but we repeat them specifically here as they have general applicability.

In certain circumstances, the algebraic expression for the estimate of the parameter of interest in a medical study may have a complex form. This complexity may, in turn, result in an even more complex expression for the corresponding standard error or in some circumstances no expression being available. In these situations, the substitution method described here may be applicable.

In some situations when the sample size is small, one may have to decide on whether the large sample expressions for the confidence interval may have to be replaced by exact methods. This leads to consideration of conservative intervals, so-called mid-P values and bootstrap methods.

In many clinical studies, multiple endpoints on each subject are often observed and these may lead to a large number of significance tests on the resulting data. The assessment of a patient's quality of life is one example of this in which each instrument may have many questions which may be repeated on several occasions over the study period. In other circumstances, there may be multiple comparisons to make, for example in a clinical trial comparing several treatments. We discuss how the corresponding test size is affected and the impact on how confidence intervals are reported.

The substitution method

As described throughout this book the most commonly used method of calculating confidence intervals involves the Normal approximation in which a multiple of the standard error is added to and subtracted from the sample value for the measure. The general expression is

$$\text{Estimate} - (z_{1-\alpha/2} \times \text{SE}) \quad \text{to} \quad \text{Estimate} + (z_{1-\alpha/2} \times \text{SE})$$

where SE is the standard error of the relevant estimate and $z_{1-\alpha/2}$ is the $100(1-\alpha)\%$ percentile of the Normal distribution from Table 18.1. Sometimes the use of the Normal approximation relates to a transformation of the measure of interest. For instance, confidence limits for the relative risk, R, described in chapter 7 are based on the limits for $\log_e R$, that is,

$$\log_e R - [z_{1-\alpha/2} \times \text{SE}(\log_e R)] \quad \text{to} \quad \log_e R + [z_{1-\alpha/2} \times \text{SE}(\log_e R)].$$

Transforming back to the original scale, by taking the exponential of these limits, gives the limits for the relative risk itself.

It is important to realise that it is the actual limits of the transformed quantity that must be back transformed and when the limits are transformed in this way the confidence limits are not symmetrical about the point estimate.

Unfortunately, however, for a number of measures used in epidemiology or clinical research, either no standard error formula is available or the formula is complex and tedious to calculate. In addition, these more complex formulae may not be implemented in computer software packages.

The substitution method is a particular approach to confidence interval estimation that can be used in some of these more difficult situations. It can replace the Normal approximation in others.[1] It is easily understood, simple to apply, makes fewer assumptions than the Normal approximation approach and is inherently more accurate. The essence of the method is to find an expression for the measure of interest as a function of a basic parameter for which confidence limits are easy to calculate. The confidence limits for the measure are then obtained by substituting the limits for this basic parameter into the formula for the measure.

Worked example: gene frequency

The following example illustrates a very simple application of the substitution method from the area of population genetics. Assuming Hardy–Weinberg equilibrium, the frequency (the proportion or percentage) of a rare recessive gene, q, in the population can be estimated[2] as the square root of the birth incidence of homozygotes, I, that is,

$$q = \sqrt{I}.$$

In this case, an approximation for the standard error of this estimate of q is available and is given by[2]

$$SE(q) = \sqrt{(1 - q^2)/4N},$$

where N is the number of births on which the birth incidence is based. This expression can then be used to calculate the large sample confidence interval in the usual way.

Seventeen cases of Wilson's disease were detected in 1 240 091 births in Ireland[3], giving a birth incidence of $I = 17/1\,240\,091 = 13\cdot71$ per million. This corresponds to a gene frequency of $q = \sqrt{0\cdot00001371} = 0\cdot0037$ or $0\cdot37\%$. Using the Normal approximation and the above expression for the standard error of q, the 95% confidence interval for the gene frequency is from $0\cdot28\%$ to $0\cdot46\%$.

To determine confidence limits for the gene frequency, q, using the substitution method, limits are obtained for the incidence rate I and substituted into the formula for q. Using the methods described in chapter 7, employing the Poisson distribution with $x = 17$ and Table 18.3, the 95% confidence limits for the incidence of Wilson's disease are $I_L = 7\cdot99$ and $I_U = 21\cdot95$ per million. Taking the square root of each of these limits gives 95% limits for q. Thus $q_L = \sqrt{0\cdot00000799} = 0\cdot0028 = 0\cdot28\%$ and $q_U = \sqrt{0\cdot00002195} = 0\cdot0047 = 0\cdot47\%$. These are almost identical to those obtained using the Normal approximation above.

The substitution method for obtaining confidence limits for the gene frequency relies on the fact that q can be expressed as the square root of the birth incidence, for which limits are readily calculated. The square root of these limits gives the confidence limits for the gene frequency.

The simplicity of the standard error formula for the gene frequency example above means that, in this case, the substitution method shows no advantage in terms of ease of use. However, the utility of the method is illustrated in the derivation of confidence limits for the incidence rate, the attributable risk (chapter 7) and the number needed to treat (chapter 11). In particular the standard error formula for the attributable risk is quite complex and the substitution limits provide a much easier method for performing the calculation.[1] Other examples of the substitution method are to be found. In particular, confidence limit estimation based on a transformation of a particular quantity, such as that described for the relative risk above, can also be considered an application of the method.

A major advantage of the substitution method is that no distributional assumptions are necessary for the sampling distribution of the measure for which the confidence limits are required. If exact confidence limits are known for the underlying parameter (as in the binomial or Poisson cases) the limits for a function of the parameter will also be exact. For example, the substitution limits described above for the gene frequency, which are based on exact limits for the incidence rate, are in general more accurate than those obtained using the standard error formula. Thus there may be a distinct advantage to the substitution method even when an alternative exists.

The kernel of the substitution method is expressing the measure for which confidence limits are required as a function of a single quantity for which limits are easily obtained. It is important to note, however, that the measure must be a function of a single parameter for the method to work. For example, it is not possible to obtain a confidence interval for a relative risk by using the confidence limits for its two component absolute risks.

To avoid multiple parameters it may be necessary to assume that some of the quantities that make up the relevant formula are without sampling variation and are thus regarded as having no variation. If the measure is derived from a contingency table this will often be equivalent to assuming that one or both of the margins of the table are fixed. Thus the substitution limits for the attributable risk (chapter 7) assume that the prevalence of the risk factor is constant and the substitution limits for an incidence rate (chapter 7) assume that the population size is fixed. This aspect has been discussed further.[4–6]

Comment

The substitution method will be applicable as long as there is a fairly simple relationship between the measure and the parameter for which limits are available. Technically, the measure must either increase or decrease as the parameter value increases. Most measures in epidemiology and clinical medicine, however, satisfy this requirement.

The substitution method for deriving confidence intervals may be useful to the researcher faced with a non-standard measure or one with a fairly complex standard error. It is particularly suitable for "hand" calculations when specialised computer software is not available.

Exact and mid-P confidence intervals

One way of thinking about confidence intervals for a population parameter, θ, is that a 95% confidence interval contains those values of θ that are not rejected by a hypothesis test at the 5% level using the observed data. As a consequence, one can determine lower and upper limits (θ_L, θ_U) as the values that are on the "exact" borderline of significance by the two possible one-sided tests both at the 2·5% level. For example, suppose we observed 50 remissions out of 100 patients, giving a response rate of 0·5. Using the traditional method of chapter 6, a 95% confidence interval for the true proportion θ is 0·4 to 0·6. Suppose the true remission rate was in fact 0·4, the lower of these limits, that is it corresponded exactly to our estimate of θ_L, then, in a trial of 100 patients we would expect to observe 50 or *more* remissions with probability of about 0·025. Similarly, if the true remission rate were 0·6 (exactly our estimate of θ_U) we would expect to observe 50 or *fewer* remissions with a probability of about 0·025. These probabilities are not precisely 0·025 because the standard deviations necessary for these calculations are based on $\theta = 0\cdot4$ and $\theta = 0\cdot6$ respectively, rather than $\theta = 0\cdot5$.

An exact confidence interval for this remission proportion would involve using the binomial distribution to calculate the probability of 50 or *more* remissions in 100 patients for a variety of possible values of the true population parameter, θ. The lower limit, θ_L, is then the value of θ which gives a probability of exactly 0·025 (hence the term "exact" confidence interval). A similar calculation provides θ_U. This process would appear to be ideal, and many textbooks recommend it. However, because of the discrete nature of count data precise correspondence with (here) 0·025 cannot often be obtained. Thus the coverage probability for an exact confidence interval tends to be larger than the nominal one of $100(1 - \alpha)\%$. So what purports to be a 95% confidence interval is actually wider, and may exclude the true population value on, say, only 3% of occasions rather than the desired 5%. For small studies an exact interval may be much wider than is desired.[7]

For small samples, instead of the usual chi-squared test, a commonly used test is *Fisher's Exact Test*.[8] For this test the data for calculating the two proportions are first expressed by placing the observations in a 2×2 table, with the total for the columns and rows known as the marginal totals. This format also provides an estimate of the odds ratio (chapter 7). Given the marginal totals, it is possible to calculate the probability of the observed table, using the so-called *hypergeometric distribution*.[8,9] Fisher's Exact Test involves calculating the probability of all the possible tables that can be constructed that have the same marginal totals as the observed one. For convenience, these tables can be ordered in terms of the odds ratios of the individual tables.

The actual observed data table has the highest probability, with the probabilities decreasing as the odds ratio moves away from the observed one in either direction. The one-sided P value is the sum of all probabilities more extreme (in a given direction) than the observed one, plus the probability of the observed table. The simplest way to derive a two-sided P value is to double the one-sided P value. It can be shown that this test is conservative, which simplistically means that the associated P value is too large. In particular, under the assumption that the null hypothesis is true the expected value of this one-sided P value is greater than 0·5, whereas it should be exactly 0·5, since under the null hypothesis one would expect the P value to be uniformly distributed over the interval 0 to 1.

An alternative is known as the mid-P value and involves adding only half (rather than all) the probability of the observed table to the sum of probabilities of the more extreme tables to obtain the one-sided P value.[8–10] Clearly this mid-P value will be smaller, and so results in a less conservative hypothesis test. It can also be shown that its expected value under the null hypothesis is 0·5. This is particularly important when the results of different studies are pooled[7] (see chapter 11). In practice, we usually deal with two-sided tests, and the two-sided mid-P value is simply double the one-sided mid-P value.[10]

The approach to confidence intervals via hypothesis tests can use mid-P probabilities rather than exact probabilities to obtain mid-P confidence intervals.[9] They are more tedious to calculate than the corresponding limits using the more conventional methods as there is no direct formula. They give narrower limits than conventional intervals, but simulations have shown for a binomial proportion that the coverage probabilities are close to the specified ones, except for values of the proportion close to 0 or 1.[7,11]

Example

Swinscow[8] compares the injury rates in two parachute dropping zones as 5 out of 15 drops in one zone and 2 out of 40 drops in another zone. The conventional two-sided Fisher's Exact Test result is P = 0·0251 and the mid-P value is 0·0136. The estimated odds ratio is

$$OR = \frac{5 \times (40 - 2)}{(15 - 5) \times 2} = 9.5$$

and a 95% confidence interval based on the probabilities from the Fisher Exact Test is 1·25 to 107·9. The mid-P 95% confidence interval is 1·54 to 75·5. This narrower confidence interval reflects the less conservative inference obtained using mid-P values. It is perhaps worth noting that the 95% confidence interval using the traditional large sample assumptions is 1·60 to 56·4, which is even narrower. However, this interval would not, in the long run, have 95% coverage of the population odds ratio because the large sample assumptions do not hold for small samples (chapter 6).

Comment

Rothman and Greenland[10] remark on the exact versus mid-P debate that "neither position is logically compelling ... the choice is of little practical importance because any data set in which the choice makes a big numerical difference must have very little information on the measure of interest". It should be noted that the coverage properties of exact and mid-P confidence intervals for more complicated situations such as the difference between binomial proportions have yet to be investigated thoroughly although Newcombe[12] has investigated their properties through simulation.

The use of the mid-P method when comparing a sample proportion with a specified population proportion is discussed by Tai *et al.*[13]

Software

Exact confidence intervals for a variety of situations are available in the StatXact 3 software (http://www.cytel.com) which also give mid-P confidence intervals for the particular case of a confidence interval for an odds ratio.

Bootstrap confidence intervals

Conventional confidence interval calculations require assumptions concerning the sampling distribution of the estimate of interest. If the sample size is large and we wish to estimate a confidence interval for a mean, then the form of the underlying population distribution is not important because the central limit theorem will ensure that the sampling distribution is approximately Normal. However, if the sample size is small we can only presume a t distribution form for the sampling distribution if the underlying population distribution can be assumed Normal. If this is not the case then the confidence interval cannot be expected to cover the population value with the specified confidence coverage, say 95%. In practice, we have information on the form of the distribution of the population from the distribution of the sample data itself. The so-called "bootstrap" estimates (from the expression "pulling oneself up by one's bootstraps") utilise this information, by making repeated random samples with replacement of the same size as the original sample from the data.[14,15] In this way the bootstrap samples mimic the way the observed data are collected from the population. The "with replacement" means that any observation can be sampled more than once. It is important because sampling without replacement would simply give the original data values in different orders with, for example, the mean and standard deviation always being exactly the same. It turns out that "with replacement" is the best approach if the observations are independent; if they are not then other methods, beyond the scope of this chapter, are needed. The standard error is estimated from the variability between the values of the statistic derived from the different bootstrap samples. The point about the bootstrap is that it produces a variety of values obtained from the observations themselves, whose variability reflects the standard error which would be obtained if samples had been repeatedly taken from the original population.

Suppose we wish to calculate a 95% confidence interval for a mean. We take a random sample of the data, of the same size as the original sample, and calculate the mean of the data in this random sample. We do this repeatedly, say 999 times. We now have 999 means. If these are ordered in increasing value a bootstrap 95% confidence interval for the mean would be from the 25th to the 975th values. This is known as the *percentile method*.

However, the percentile method is not the best method of bootstrapping because it can have a bias, which one can estimate and correct for using methods, such as the "bias corrected method" and the "bias corrected and accelerated" (BCa) method, the latter being the preferred option. There is also the "parametric bootstrap" when the residuals from a parametric model are boot-strapped to give estimates of the standard errors of the parameters, for example to estimate the standard errors of coefficients from a multiple regression. Details are given in Efron and Tibshirani[14] or Davison and Hinckley.[15]

Using the methods above, valid bootstrap confidence intervals can be constructed for all common estimators, such as a proportion, a median, or a difference in means, providing that the data are independent and come from the same population. More sophisticated methods can also allow for correlations between the observations.

The number of bootstrap samples required depends on the type of estimator: 50–200 are adequate for a confidence interval for a mean, but in excess of 1000 replications are required for a confidence interval of, say, the 2·5% or 97·5% centiles. When quoting a bootstrap confidence interval one should state the method, such as the percentile or bias corrected, and the number of replications used.

Worked example

Consider the β-endorphin concentrations from 11 runners described in chapter 5. One method of calculating a confidence interval for a median is described there. To calculate a 95% confidence interval for the median using a bootstrap approach we first decide on the number of replications (say 999), generate the samples and calculate from each the median as Table 13.1.

The 999 bootstrap medians are then ordered by increasing value. The 25th and the 975th values give the percentile estimates of the 95% confidence interval. In this example, we find that the BCa method gives a 95% bootstrap confidence interval 71·2 to 143·0 pmol/l. This contrasts with 71·2 to 177·0 pmol/l using the standard method given in chapter 5. The bootstrap interval suggests that the lower limit from the standard method is probably about right but the upper limit may be too high.

Table 13.1 Summary of 999 bootstrap samples from 11 observations of β-endorphin concentrations in pmol/l[16]

	β-endorphin concentrations in pmol/l	Median
Original data	66, 71·2, 83·0, 83·6, 101, 107·6, 122, 143, 160, 177, 414	107·6
Bootstrap:		
Sample 1	143, 107·6, 414, 160, 101, 177, 107·6, 160, 160, 160, 101	160
Sample 2	122, 414, 101, 83·6, 143, 107·6, 101, 143, 143, 143, 107·6	122
. . .	. . .	. . .
Sample 999	122, 414, 160, 177, 101, 107·6, 83·6, 177, 177, 107·6, 107·6	122

When the standard and the bootstrap methods agree, we can be more confident about the inference we are making and this is an important use of the bootstrap. When they disagree more caution is needed, but the relatively simple assumptions required by the bootstrap method for validity imply that, in general, it is to be preferred.

It may seem that the best estimator of the median for the population is the median of the bootstrap estimates, but this turns out not to be the case. One should quote the sample median, here 107·6 pmol/l, as the best estimate of the population median.

The main advantage of the bootstrap is that it frees the investigator from making inappropriate assumptions about the distribution of an estimator in order to make inferences. A particular advantage is that it is available when the formula for the confidence interval cannot be derived explicitly and it may provide better estimates when the formulae are only approximate.

Comment

The naïve bootstrap methods we have described make the assumption that the observed data sample is an unbiased simple random sample from the study population. More complex survey sampling schemes, such as stratified random sampling, may not reflect this simple situation, and so more complicated bootstrapping schemes may be required. Naïve bootstrapping may not be successful in very small samples (say <9 observations), since the observations themselves are less likely to be representative of the study population. "In very small samples even a badly fitting parametric analysis may outperform a non-parametric analysis, by providing less variable results at the expense of a tolerable amount of bias."[14]

Perhaps one of the most common uses for bootstrapping in medical research has been for calculating confidence intervals for derived statistics such as cost-effectiveness ratios, when the theoretical distribution is mathematically difficult.[17,18] However, care is needed here since the denominators in some bootstrap samples can get close to zero, leading to very large estimates of the ratio. As an example in health economics, Lambert et al.[19] calculated the mean resource costs per patient for day patients with active rheumatoid arthritis as £1789 with a bootstrap 95% confidence interval of £1539 to £2027 (1000 replications). They used a bootstrap method because the resource costs have a very skewed distribution.

However, the authors did not state which bootstrap method they used.

Software

It is relatively easy to program the bootstrap with modern software. Three packages which have the bootstrap as standard are Stata (http://www.stata.com), SPlus (http://www.mathsoft.com) and Resampling Stats (http://www.resample.com). The book by Davison and Hinckley[15] comes with a disk of software and examples for use with SPlus. The results in this chapter were derived using SPlus.

Multiple comparisons

In a clinical study in which two groups are being compared, the formal statistical test of this comparison has an associated two-sided test 'size' of α. This is set as the boundary below which the P value, calculated from the data for the primary endpoint of the study, must fall to be declared statistically significant. In this case the null hypothesis of no difference between groups is then rejected. We have argued very strongly against the uncritical use of such an approach (chapter 3) but introduce it here for illustrative purposes.

Suppose this approach is utilised in the analysis of a clinical trial comparing two groups and suppose further that there is truly no difference between the two groups. Despite this "no difference" there is a $100\alpha\%$ probability of a statistically significant result and the false rejection of the null hypothesis. Thus, following any comparison, there is always the possibility of a false positive outcome. It is usual to set this probability as 5% (i.e., $\alpha = 0.05$).

If more than one endpoint is measured for the two group study in question, then the situation becomes more complex. For example, if a clinical trial is comparing two treatments (A and B) but there are three different independent outcomes being measured, then there are three comparisons to make between A and B and, in theory at least, three statistical tests. In this circumstance it can be shown that the false-positive rate is no longer $100\alpha\%$ but approximately $300\alpha\%$. In fact for k (assumed independent) outcome measures the false-positive rate is $100 \times [1 - (1 - \alpha)^k]\%$ which is approximately equal to $100k\alpha\%$. Clearly, the false-positive rate increases as the number of comparisons increases.

In order to retain the false-positive rate as $100\alpha\%$ the *Bonferroni correction* is often suggested. This implies declaring differences as statistically significant at the $100\alpha\%$ only if the observed P is less than α/k. In the case of $\alpha = 0.05$ and $k = 3$, this implies P < 0.017. Equivalently, and preferably, multiply the observed P value by k and declare this significant if less than α. This latter approach is recommended by Altman[20] as it avoids the apparently anomalous situation in which the P value quoted is less than α but is *not* statistically significant.

Similar considerations can apply to confidence intervals and one approach in situations where k endpoints are being compared is to replace $z_{1-\alpha/2}$ in the corresponding equation for the confidence interval by $z_{1-\alpha/2k}$. For example, if $k = 3$, $\alpha = 0.05$, then $z_{1-\alpha/2} = z_{0.975} = 1.96$ is replaced by $z_{1-\alpha/2k} = z_{0.9917} = 2.64$ (see Table 18.1). This approach clearly leads to a wider confidence interval. (Analogous changes would be made if t rather than z were being used for constructing the confidence interval.)

Worked example

Suppose in the first worked example of chapter 4 that both the systolic and diastolic blood pressures were measured. Thus the study has $k = 2$ endpoints. In this case to calculate the 95% confidence interval corresponding to the observed mean systolic blood pressure of 146.4 mmHg (SD 18.5) we utilise $\alpha/2 = 0.025$ in place of $\alpha = 0.05$ to obtain from Table 18.1 $z_{1-\alpha/4} = z_{0.9875} = 2.24$. The 95% confidence interval for the population value of the mean systolic blood pressure is then given by

$$146.4 - (2.24 \times 1.85) \quad \text{to} \quad 146.4 + (2.24 \times 1.85)$$

that is, from 142.3 to 150.5 mmHg. (This compares with 142.7 to 150.1 mmHg in chapter 4.) In addition we would calculate the 95% confidence interval for the diastolic blood pressure also using 2.24 in place of 1.96 in the calculation.

It is recognised that the Bonferroni approach to adjusting for multiple comparisons is conservative as it assumes the different endpoints are uncorrelated. Indeed, in the example we are using, it is well known that systolic and diastolic blood pressures are strongly correlated. This conservativeness implies that utilising the criterion $kP < \alpha$ will lead to failure to reject the null hypothesis on too many occasions. The corresponding confidence intervals will also be too wide. However, the correlation structure between different endpoints measured on the same subjects may be very complex and not easily summarised or corrected for and, in any event, will change from study to study.

One approach that has been used to overcome this difficulty is to quote 99% confidence intervals rather than 95% confidence intervals when more than a single outcome is regarded as primary. Thus the UK Prospective Diabetes Study Group[21] report 21 distinct endpoints, ranging from fatal myocardial infarction to death from unknown cause, and provide 99% confidence intervals for the corresponding 21 relative risks comparing tight with less tight control of blood pressure. This is a "half-way house" proposal, since $0.01 \, (= 1 - 0.99)$ is between the conventional 0.05 and the Bonferroni corrected value of $0.05/21 = 0.0024$.

A contrary view warning against the indiscriminate use of the Bonferroni correction, points out that the method is concerned with the situation that all k null hypotheses are true simultaneously, which is rarely of interest or use to researchers.[22,23] A further weakness is that the interpretation of a finding depends on the number of other tests performed. Thus two investigators obtaining exactly the same result with a particular endpoint may draw different conclusions on statistical significance if they had observed a different number of other endpoints. In general there is also an increasing likelihood that truly important differences are deemed non-significant.

There are other situations in which multiple comparisons may be made. For example, in the meta-analyses described in chapter 11, many independent trial results may be summarised by their individual treatment effects and associated 95% confidence intervals before combining into a single summary estimate with a confidence interval. A more cautious approach would be to utilise 99% confidence intervals in their place.

Similar considerations of multiplicity may also apply in situations other than studies with multiple endpoints. For example, if more than two groups are compared in a clinical trial using a single outcome, then there is potentially more than one statistical test to conduct and more than one confidence interval to construct.

There are also situations in which a multiple comparison approach is utilised to compare different groups inappropriately. For example, Rothman[24] illustrated, using data from Young et al.,[25] how subjects from four groups are compared and are not statistically significantly different from each other using a test size of 5% without a Bonferroni correction. However, he points out that there is some structure to the four groups that had not been taken into account in this analysis. The four groups were in fact four levels of water chlorination: none, low, medium and high. Taking this "dose" into account with a suitable test for trend demonstrated a statistically significant and increasing relative risk of brain cancer amongst the women under study with increasing dose. (See also the example of multiple logistic regression in chapter 8.)

Multiple comparisons can also occur in continuous monitoring of the progress of clinical trials which include interim analyses, subgroup analyses in trials and other studies, and in regression modelling when decisions on inclusion and exclusion of variables in a model have to be made. All of these have direct implications for the corresponding confidence intervals.

Comment

As we have indicated, the problem of multiple comparisons is particularly acute in quality of life research. Thus published guidelines on reporting such studies explicitly state: "in the case of multiple comparisons, attention must be paid to the total number of comparisons, to the adjustment, if any, of the significance level, and to the interpretation of the results".[26] Improved, but more complex, methods of correcting for multiple comparisons are available and their relative merits have been discussed.[27] There is no general consensus, however, as to which procedures to adopt to allow for multiple comparisons. We therefore recommend reporting the unadjusted P values and confidence limits with a suitable note of caution with respect to interpretation. Perneger[23] concludes that: "Simply describing what tests of significance have been performed, and why, is generally the best way of dealing with multiple comparisons." A precautionary recommendation may be to follow the UK Prospective Diabetes Study Group[21] and at least have in mind a 99% confidence interval as an aid to interpretation.

1 Daly LE. Confidence limits made easy: Interval estimation using a substitution method. *Am J Epidemiol* 1998;**147**:783–90.

2 Weir, BS. *Genetic data analysis II*. Sunderland, Massachusetts: Sinauer Associates, 1996.

3 Reilly M, Daly L, Hutchinson M. An epidemiological study of Wilson's disease in the Republic of Ireland. *J Neurol Neurosurg Psychiat* 1993;**56**:298–300.

4 Greenland S. Re: "Confidence limits made easy: Interval estimation using a substitution method". *Am J Epidemiol* 1999;**149**:884.

5 Newcombe RG. Re: "Confidence limits made easy: Interval estimation using a substitution method". *Am J Epidemiol* 1999;**149**:884–5.

6 Daly LE. Re: "Confidence limits made easy: Interval estimation using a substitution method" [author's reply]. *Am J Epidemiol* 1999;**149**:885–6.

7 Agresti A, Coull BA. Approximate is better than "exact" for interval estimation of binomial proportions. *Am Stat* 1998;**52**:119–26.

8 Swinscow TDV. *Statistics at square one*. 9th ed revised by MJ Campbell. London: British Medical Association, 1996.

9 Berry G, Armitage P. Mid-P confidence intervals: a brief review. *Statistician* 1995;**44**:417–23.

10 Rothman KJ, Greenland S. *Modern epidemiology*. 2nd ed. Philadelphia: Lippincott-Raven, 1998.

11 Vollset SE. Confidence intervals for a binomial proportion. *Stat Med* 1993;**12**:809–24.

12 Newcombe RG. Interval estimation for the difference between independent proportions: Comparison of eleven methods. *Stat Med* 1998;**17**:873–90.

13 Tai B-C, Lee J, Lee H-P. Comparing a sample proportion with a specified proportion based on the mid-P method. *Psychiatry Res* 1997;**71**:201–3.

14 Efron B, Tibshirani RJ. *An introduction to the bootstrap*. New York: Chapman and Hall, 1993.

15 Davison A, Hinckley D. *Bootstrap methods and their applications*. Cambridge: Cambridge University Press, 1997.

16 Dale G, Fleetwood JA, Weddell A, Ellis RD, Sainsbury JRC. β-Endorphin: a factor in "fun run" collapse. *BMJ* 1987;**294**:1004.

17 Campbell MK, Torgerson D. Confidence intervals for cost-effectiveness ratios: the use of "bootstrapping". *J Health Services Res Policy* 1997;**2**:253–5.

18 Chaudhary MA, Stearns SC. Estimating confidence intervals for cost-effectiveness ratios: an example from a randomized trial. *Stat Med* 1996;**15**:1447–58.

19 Lambert CM, Hurst NP, Forbes JF, Lochhead A, Macleod M, Nuki G. Is day care equivalent to inpatient care for active rheumatoid arthritis? Randomised controlled clinical and economic evaluation. *BMJ* 1998;**316**:965–9.

20 Altman DG. *Practical statistics for medical research*. London: Chapman and Hall, 1991:210–12.

21 UK Prospective Diabetes Study Group. Tight blood pressure control and risk of macrovascular and microvascular complications in type 2 diabetes: UKPDS 38. *BMJ* 1998;**317**:703–12.

22 Rothman KJ. No adjustments are needed for multiple comparisons. *Epidemiology* 1990;**1**:43–6.

23 Perneger TV. What's wrong with Bonferroni adjustments. *BMJ* 1998;**316**: 1236–8.

24 Rothman KJ. *Modern epidemiology*. Boston: Little, Brown, 1986: figure 16.2.

25 Young TB, Kanarek MS, Tsiatis AA. Epidemiologic study of drinking water chlorination and Wisconsin female cancer mortality. *J Natl Cancer Inst* 1981; **67**:1191–8.

26 Staquet MJ, Berzon RA, Osoba D, Machin D. Guidelines for reporting results of quality of life assessments in clinical trials. *Quality Life Res* 1996;**5**:496–502.

27 Sankoh AJ, Huque MF, Dubin SD. Some comments on frequently used multiple endpoint adjustment methods in clinical trials. *Stat Med* 1997;**16**:2529-42.

Part II
Statistical guidelines and checklists

14 Statistical guidelines for contributors to medical journals

DOUGLAS G ALTMAN, SHEILA M GORE,
MARTIN J GARDNER, STUART J POCOCK

Introduction

Most papers published in medical journals contain analyses that
have been carried out without any help from a statistician.
Although nearly all medical researchers have some acquaintance
with basic statistics, there is no easy way for them to acquire
insight into important statistical concepts and principles. There
is also little help available about how to design, analyse, and
write up a whole project. Partly for these reasons much that is published in medical journals is statistically poor or even wrong.[1] A
high level of statistical errors has been noted in several reviews
of journal articles and has caused much concern.[2,3]

Few journals offer even rudimentary statistical advice to contributors. These guidelines (originally published in 1983) followed
suggestions[1,4] that comprehensive statistical guidelines could
help by making medical researchers more aware of important
statistical principles, and by indicating what information ought
to be supplied in a paper. Since our original article, Bailar and
Mosteller published guidelines amplifying the brief section on
statistics in the "Uniform requirements for manuscripts".[5,6]
Other authors have since published guidelines for particular
types of study.[7-12] Lang and Secic have published very comprehensive guidance.[13]

Deciding what to include in the guidelines, how much detail to
give, and how to deal with topics where there is no consensus was
problematic. These guidelines should thus be seen as one view
of what is important, rather than as a definitive document. We
did not set out to provide a set of rules but rather to give general
information and advice about important aspects of statistical

171

design, analysis, and presentation. Those specific recommendations that we have made are mostly strong advice against certain practices.

Some familiarity with statistical methods and ideas is assumed, since some knowledge of statistics is necessary before carrying out statistical analyses. For those with only a limited acquaintance with statistics, the guidelines should show that the subject is very much wider than mere significance testing and illustrate how important correct interpretation is. The lack of precise recommendations in some places indicates that good statistical analysis requires common sense and judgement, as well as a repertoire of formal techniques, so that there is an art in statistics as well as in medicine. We hope that the guidelines present an uncontroversial view of the most frequently used and accepted statistical procedures. We have deliberately limited the scope of the guidelines to cover the more common statistical procedures. The version presented here incorporates a few additions to the original version.

Readers may find that a relevant section presents information or advice that is unfamiliar or is not understood. In such circumstances, although almost all of the topics covered may be found in the more comprehensive medical statistics textbooks,[14-19] we strongly recommend that they should seek the advice of a statistician. The absence from the guidelines of specific references is intentional: it is better to get expert personal advice if further insight is needed. Moreover, because mistakes in design cannot later be rectified, professional advice should first be obtained when planning a research project rather than when analysing the data.

These guidelines are intended to try to help authors know what is important statistically and how to present it in their papers. They emphasise that such matters of presentation are closely linked to more general consideration of statistical principles. Detailed discussion of how to choose an appropriate statistical method is not given; such information is best obtained by consulting a statistician. We do, however, draw attention to certain misuses of statistical methods.

These guidelines follow the usual structure of medical research papers: Methods, Results (analysis and presentation), and Discussion (interpretation). As a result, several topics appear in more than one place and are cross-referenced as appropriate. Statistical checklists (chapter 15) indicate the broad categories of information that should be included in a paper.

Methods section

General principles

It is most important to describe clearly what was done, including the design of the research (be it an experiment, trial, or survey) and the collection of the data. The aim should be to give enough information to allow methods to be fully understood and, if desired, repeated by others. As noted by the International Committee of Medical Journal Editors, authors should "describe statistical methods with enough detail to enable a knowledgeable reader with access to the original data to verify the reported results".[6]

Authors should include information on the following aspects of the design of their research:

- the objective of the research, and major hypotheses;
- the type of subjects, stating criteria for inclusion and exclusion;
- the source of the subjects and how they were selected;
- the number of subjects studied and why that number of subjects was used;
- the types of observation and the measurement techniques used (where several assessments are made for each subject, the main focus of interest should be specified).

Each type of study—for example, surveys and clinical trials—will require certain additional information.

Surveys (observational studies)

The study design should be clearly explained. For instance, the selection of a control group and any matching procedures need detailed description. It should also be clearly stated whether the study is retrospective, cross-sectional, or prospective. The procedure for selecting subjects and the achievement of a high participation rate are particularly important, as findings are usually extrapolated from the sample to some general population. It is helpful to report any steps taken to encourage participation in the survey.

Clinical trials

The treatment regimens (including ancillary patient care and criteria for modifying or stopping treatment) need detailed definition. The method for allocating treatments to subjects should be stated explicitly. In particular, the specific method of randomisation (including any stratification) and how it was implemented need to be explained. Lack of randomisation should be noted as a deficiency in design and the reasons given. Studies using deterministic allocation methods, for example based on hospital number or alteration, are not truly randomised and are unlikely to be acceptable to the BMJ^{20} or other leading medical journals.

The use of blinding techniques and other precautions taken to ensure an unbiased evaluation of patient response should be described. The main criteria for comparing treatments, as agreed in the trial protocol, should be listed. For crossover trials the precise pattern of treatments (and any run in and wash out periods) needs explaining.

A more comprehensive list of information to include in the report of a clinical trial is given in the checklist in chapter 15. Many leading medical journals now require authors to comply with the CONSORT recommendations for reporting controlled trials.[12]

Statistical methods

All the statistical methods used in a paper should be identified. When several techniques are used it should be absolutely clear which method was used where, and this may need clarification in the results section. Common techniques, such as t tests, simple χ^2 tests, Wilcoxon and Mann–Whitney tests, correlation (r), and linear regression, do not need to be described, but methods with more than one form, such as t tests (paired or unpaired), analysis of variance, and rank correlation, should be identified unambiguously. More complex methods do need some explanation, and if the methods are unusual a precise reference should be given, preferably to a textbook (with page numbers). It may help to include brief comments on why the particular method of analysis was used, especially when a more familiar approach has been avoided. It is useful to give the name of a computer program or package used—for example, the Statistical Package for the Social Sciences (SPSS)—but the specific statistical methods must still be identified.

Results section: statistical analysis

Descriptive information

Adequate description of the data should precede and complement formal statistical analysis. In general variables which are important for the validity and interpretation of subsequent statistical analyses should be described in most detail. This can be achieved by graphical methods, such as scatter plots or histograms, or by using summary statistics. Continuous variables (such as weight or blood pressure) can be summarised using the mean and standard deviation (SD) or the median and a percentile range—say, the interquartile range (25th to 75th percentile). The latter approach is preferable when continuous measurements have an asymmetrical distribution. The standard error (SE) is not appropriate for describing variability. For ordered qualitative data (such as stages of disease I to IV) the calculation of means and standard deviations is incorrect; instead, proportions should be reported.

Deviations from the intended study design should be described. For example, in clinical trials it is particularly important to enumerate withdrawals with reasons, if known, and treatment allocation. For surveys, where the response rate is of fundamental importance, it is valuable to give information on the characteristics of the non-responders compared with those who took part. The representativeness of the study sample will need to be investigated if it is a prime intention to extrapolate results to some appropriate population.

It is useful to compare the distribution of baseline characteristics in different groups, such as treatment groups in a randomised trial. Such differences that exist, even if not statistically significant, are real and should be properly allowed for in the analysis (see "Complex analyses", below). Such tests assess only the integrity of the randomisation, not whether the groups are comparable.

Underlying assumptions

Methods of analysis such as *t* tests, correlation, regression, and analysis of variance all depend to some extent on certain assumptions about the distribution of the variable(s) being analysed. Technically, these assumptions are that in some aspect the data come from a Normal distribution and if two or more groups are being compared that the variability within each is the same.

It is not possible to give absolutely the degree to which these assumptions may be violated without invalidating the analysis. But data which have a highly skewed (asymmetrical) distribution or for which the variability is considerably different across groups may require either some transformation before analysis (see "Data transformation", below) or the use of alternative

175

"distribution free" methods, which do not depend on assumptions about the distribution (often called non-parametric methods). For example, the Mann–Whitney U test is the distribution free equivalent of the two-sample t test. Distribution-free methods may also be appropriate for small data sets, for which the assumptions cannot be validated adequately.

Sometimes the assumption of Normality may be especially important—for example, when the range of values calculated as two standard deviations either side of the mean is taken as a 95% "normal range" or reference interval. In such cases the distributional assumption must be shown to be justified.

Hypothesis tests

The main purpose of hypothesis tests (often less accurately referred to as "significance tests") is to evaluate a limited number of preformulated hypotheses. Other tests, which are carried out because they have been suggested by preliminary inspection of the data, will give a false impression because in such circumstances the calculated P value is too small. For example, it is not valid to test the difference between the smallest and largest of a set of several means or proportions without making due allowance for the reason for testing that particular difference; special "multiple comparison" techniques are available for making pairwise comparisons among several groups. However, where three or more groups are compared which have a natural ordering, such as age groups or stages of cancer, the data should be analysed by a method that specifically evaluates a trend across groups.

It is customary to carry out two-sided hypothesis tests. If a one-sided test is used this should be indicated and justified for the problem in hand.

The presentation and interpretation of results of hypothesis tests are discussed in later sections. The use of confidence intervals in addition to hypothesis tests is strongly recommended—see next section and chapters 1 and 3.

Confidence intervals

Most studies are concerned with estimating some quantity, such as a mean difference or a relative risk. It is desirable to calculate the confidence interval around such an estimate. This is a range of values about which we are, say, 95% confident that it includes the true value. There is a close relation between the results of a test of a hypothesis and the associated confidence interval: if the difference between groups is significant at the 5% level then the associated 95% confidence interval excludes the zero difference. The confidence interval conveys more information because it indicates a range of values for the true effect which is compatible with the sample observations (see also "Interpretation of hypothesis tests", below, and chapter 3).

Confidence intervals reveal the precision of an estimate. A wide confidence interval points to lack of information, whether the difference is statistically significant or not, and is a warning against overinterpreting results from small studies.

In a comparative study, confidence intervals should be reported for the differences between groups, not for the results of each group separately.

Paired observations

It is essential to distinguish the case of unpaired observations, where the comparison is between measurements for two different groups—for example, subjects receiving alternative treatments—from that of paired observations, where the comparison is between two measurements made on the same individuals in different circumstances (such as before and after treatment). For example, where with unpaired data the two sample t test would be used, with paired data the paired t test should be used instead. Similarly, the Mann–Whitney U test for unpaired data is replaced by the paired Wilcoxon test, and the usual χ^2 test for 2×2 tables is replaced by McNemar's test. It should always be made clear which form of test was used. Likewise the method for calculating a confidence interval differs from that for unpaired observations (see chapters 4, 5, 6, and 7).

The same distinction must be made when there are three or more sets of observations. All of the statistical methods mentioned in this section may be generalised to more than two groups; in particular, paired and two-sample t tests generalise to different forms of analysis of variance.

Units of analysis

Often several measurements are made on the same patient, but the focus of interest usually remains the patient. The simplest case is when researchers study a part of the human anatomy

177

which is in duplicate, such as eyes, but sometimes very many measurements can be taken on a single patient. Multiple counting of individual patients can lead to seriously distorted results. In particular, it inflates the sample size and may lead to spurious statistical significance. The patient is the unit of investigation and thus should be the *unit of analysis*. (A related issue is discussed in the following section.)

By contrast, groups are sometimes the focus of interest. For example, in a "cluster" randomised trial groups such as hospital wards or general practices may be randomised to different interventions. In such studies it is wrong to analyse data for individual patients as if they were independent observations. Here the cluster is the correct unit of analysis.

Repeated measurements

A common study design entails recording serial measurements of the same variable(s) on the same individual at several points in time. Such data are often analysed by calculating means and standard deviations at each time and presented graphically by a line joining these means. The shape of this mean curve may not give a good idea of the shapes of the individual curves. Unless the individual responses are very similar it may be more valuable to analyse some characteristic of the individual profiles, such as the time taken to reach a peak or the length of time above a given level. This would also help to avoid the problems associated with multiple hypothesis testing (see "Many hypothesis tests", below).

Repeated measurements of the same variable on one individual under the same experimental conditions, known as *replicate readings*, should not be treated as independent observations when comparing groups of individuals. Where the number of replicates is the same for all subjects analysis is not difficult; in particular, analysis of variance is used where t tests would have been applied to unreplicated data. If the number of replicates varies among individuals, a full analysis can be very complex. The use of the largest or smallest of a series of measurements (such as maximum blood pressure during pregnancy) may be misleading if the number of observations varies widely among individuals.

Data transformation

Many biomedical variables have distributions which are positively skewed, with some very high values, and they may require mathematical transformation to make the data appropriate for analysis. In such circumstances the logarithmic (log) transformation is often applicable, although occasionally other transformations (such as square root or reciprocal) may be more suitable.

After analysis it is desirable to convert the results back into the original scale for reporting. In the common case of log transformation, the antilog of the mean of the log data (known as the "geometric mean") should be used. The standard deviation or standard error must not be antilogged, however; instead, confidence limits on the log scale can be antilogged to give a confidence interval on the original scale. A similar procedure is adopted with other transformations when there is a single sample, but back transformation of the confidence limits for a difference between sample means makes sense only for the log transformation (see chapter 4).

If a transformation is used it is important to check that the desired effect (such as an approximately Normal distribution) is achieved. It should not be assumed that the log transformation, for instance, is necessarily suitable for all positively skewed variables.

Outliers

Observations that are highly inconsistent with the main body of the data should not be excluded from the analysis unless there are additional reasons to doubt their credibility. Any omission of such outliers should be reported. Because outliers can have a pronounced effect on a statistical analysis, it can be useful to analyse the data both with and without such observations to assess how much any conclusions depend on these values.

Correlation

It is preferable to include a scatter plot of the data for each correlation coefficient presented, although this may not be possible if there are several variables. When many variables are being investigated it is useful to show the correlations between all pairs of variables in a table (correlation matrix), rather than quoting just the largest or significant values.

For data which are irregularly distributed the rank correlation can be calculated instead of the usual Pearson "product moment" correlation (r). Rank correlation can also be used for variables that are constrained to be above or below certain values—for example, birth weights below 2500 g—or for ordered categorical variables. Rank correlation is also preferable when the relation between the variables is not linear, or when the values of one variable have been chosen by the experimenter rather than being unconstrained.

The correlation coefficient is a useful summary of the degree of linear association between two quantitative variables, but it is one of the most misused statistical methods. There are several circumstances in which correlation ought not to be used. It is incorrect to calculate a simple correlation coefficient for data which include more than one observation on some or all of the subjects, because such observations are not independent. Correlation is inappropriate for comparing alternative methods of measurement of the same variable because it assesses association, not agreement. The use of correlation to relate change over time to the initial value can give grossly misleading results.

It may be misleading to calculate the correlation coefficient for data comprising subgroups known to differ in their mean levels of one or both variables—for example, combining data for men and women when one of the variables is height.

Regression and correlation are separate techniques serving different purposes and need not automatically accompany each other. The interpretation of correlation coefficients is discussed below ("Association and causality").

Regression

It is highly desirable to present a fitted regression line together with a scatter diagram of the raw data. A plot of the fitted line without the data gives little further information than the regression equation itself. It is useful to give the values of the slope (with its standard error) and intercept and a measure of the scatter of the points around the fitted line (the residual standard deviation). A confidence interval may be constructed for a regression line and prediction intervals for individuals based on the fitted relationship. The lines joining these values are not parallel to the regression line but curved, showing the greater uncertainty of the prediction corresponding to values on the horizontal (x) axis away from the bulk of the observations (see chapter 8).

Regression on data including distinct subgroups can give misleading results, particularly if the groups differ in their mean level of the dependent (y) variable. More reliable results may be obtained by using analysis of covariance (see chapter 8).

Regression and correlation are separate techniques serving different purposes and need not automatically accompany each other. The interpretation of regression analysis is discussed below ("Prediction and diagnostic tests").

Survival data

The reporting of survival data should include graphical or tabular presentation of life tables, with details of how many patients were at risk (of dying, say) at different follow up times (see chapter 9). The life table or actuarial survival curve deals efficiently with the "censored" survival times which arise when patients are lost to follow up or are still alive; their survival time is known to be only at least so many days. To avoid misinterpretation of the unreliable later part of the curve, it may help to truncate the survival curve when there are only a few (say five) subjects still at risk. The calculation of mean survival time is inadvisable in the presence of censoring and because the distribution of survival times is usually positively skewed.

Comparison between treatment groups of the proportion surviving at arbitrary fixed times can be misleading and is generally less efficient than the comparison of life tables by a method such as the logrank test. Methods for calculating estimates of survival and confidence intervals are given in chapter 9.

When there are sufficient deaths one can show how the risk of dying varies with time by plotting, for suitable equal time intervals, the proportion of those alive at the beginning of each time interval who died during that interval. Adjusting for patient factors which might influence prognosis is possible using regression models appropriate to survival data (see next section).

Comparison of survival between the group of individuals who respond to treatment and the group who do not is misleading and should never be performed.

Complex analyses

In many studies the observations of prime interest may be influenced by several other variables. These might be anything that varies among subjects and which might have affected the outcome being observed. For example, in clinical trials they might include patient characteristics or signs and symptoms. Some or all of the covariates can be combined by appropriate multiple regression techniques to explain or predict an outcome variable, be it a continuous variable (blood pressure), a qualitative variable (post-operative thrombosis), or the length of survival (using, respectively, multiple linear regression, multiple logistic regression, or proportional hazards (Cox) regression analysis). Even in randomised clinical trials investigators may need assurance that the treatment effect is still present after simultaneous adjustment for several risk factors. When models are used to obtain estimates adjusted for other variables, it should be made clear which variables were adjusted for, on what basis they were selected, and, if relevant, how continuous variables were treated in the analysis.

Multivariate techniques, for dealing with more than one outcome variable simultaneously, really require expert help and are beyond the scope of these guidelines. Any complex statistical methods should be communicated in a manner that is comprehensible to the reader. It may help to place technical material in an appendix.

Results section: presentation of results

Presentation of summary statistics

Mean values should not be quoted without some measure of variability or precision. The standard deviation (SD) should be used to show the variability among individuals and the standard error of the mean (SE) to show the precision of the sample mean (see chapter 3: appendix 1). It must be made clear which is presented.

The use of the symbol $\pm$ to attach the standard error or standard deviation to the mean (as in 14.2 ± 1.9) causes confusion and should be avoided. Several medical journals do not now allow its use. The presentation of means as, for example, 14·2 (SE 1·9) or 14·2 (SD 7·4) is preferable. Confidence intervals are a good way of providing a reasonable indication of uncertainty of sample means, proportions, and other statistics. For example, a 95% confidence interval for the true mean is from about two standard errors below the observed mean to two standard errors above it (see chapter 4). Confidence intervals are more clearly presented as 10·4 to 18·0 (see chapter 3) than by use of the $\pm$ symbol.

When paired comparisons are made, such as when using paired t tests, it is important to give the mean and standard deviation of the differences between the observations or the standard error of the mean difference as appropriate (see chapter 3: appendix 1).

For data that have been analysed with distribution free methods it is more appropriate to give the median and a central range, covering, for example, 95% of the observations, than to use the mean and standard deviation (see "Descriptive information", above). Non-parametric confidence intervals can be calculated (see chapter 5). Likewise, if analysis has been carried out on transformed data, the mean and standard deviation of the raw data will probably not be good measures of the centre and spread of the data and should not be presented.

When percentages are given, the denominator should always be made clear. For small samples, the use of percentages is unhelpful. When percentages are contrasted it is important to distinguish an absolute difference from a relative difference. For example, a reduction from 25% to 20% may be expressed as either 5% or 20%.

Results for individuals

The overall range is not a good indicator of the variability of a set of observations as it can be strongly affected by a single extreme value and it increases with sample size. If the data have a reasonably Normal distribution the interval two standard deviations either side of the mean will cover about 95% of the observations, but a percentile range is more widely applicable to other distributions (see "Descriptive information", above).

Although statistical analysis is concerned with average effects, in many circumstances it is important also to consider how individual subjects responded. Thus, for example, it is very often clinically relevant to know how many patients did not improve with a treatment as well as the average benefit. An average effect should not be interpreted as applying to all individuals (see also "Repeated measurements", above).

Presentation of results of hypothesis tests

Hypothesis tests yield observed values of test statistics which are compared with tabulated values for the appropriate distribution (Normal, t, χ^2 etc.) to derive associated P values. It is desirable to report the observed values of the test statistics and not just the P values. The quantitative results being tested, such as mean values, proportions, correlation coefficients, should be given whether the test was significant or not. It should be made clear precisely which data have been analysed. If symbols, such as asterisks, are used to denote levels of probability, these must be defined and it is helpful if they are the same throughout the paper.

183

P values are conventionally given as <0.05, <0.01, or <0.001, but there is no reason other than familiarity for using these particular values. Exact P values (to no more than two significant figures), such as $P = 0.18$ or 0.03, are more helpful. It is unlikely to be necessary to specify levels of P lower than 0.0001. Calling any value with $P > 0.05$ "not significant" is not recommended, as it may obscure results that are not quite statistically significant but do suggest a real effect (see "Interpretation of hypothesis tests", below). When quoting P values it is important to distinguish $<$ (less than) from $>$ (greater than). P values between two limits should be expressed in logical order—for example, $0.01 < P < 0.05$ where P lies between 0.01 and 0.05. P values given in tables need not be repeated in the text.

The interpretation of hypothesis tests and P values is discussed below ("Interpretation of hypothesis tests").

Figures (graphical presentation)

Graphical display of results is helpful to readers, and figures that show individual observations are to be encouraged. Points on a graph relating to the same individual on different occasions should preferably be joined, or symbols used to indicate the related points. A helpful alternative is to plot the difference between occasions for each individual.

The customary "error bars" of one standard error above and below the mean depict only a 67% confidence interval, and are thus liable to misinterpretation; 95% confidence intervals are preferable. The presentation of such information in figures is subject to the same considerations as discussed above ("Presentation of summary statistics"). Figures are most valuable when they display data that are too complex to put into a table. At the other extreme, a figure that displays, say, only two or three means with their standard errors or confidence intervals is often a waste of space; either more information should be added, such as the raw data, or the summary values should be put in the text or a table instead. Tables are also preferable if the data values are likely to be used by others in subsequent analyses (including meta-analysis).

Scatter diagrams relating two variables should show all the observations, even if this means slight adjustment to accommodate duplicate points. These may also be indicated by replacing the plotting symbol by the actual number of coincident points.

Tables

It is much easier to scan numerical results down columns rather than across rows, and so it is better to have different types of information (such as means and standard errors) in separate columns. The number of observations should be stated for each result in a table. Tables giving information about individual patients, geographical areas, and so on are easier to read if the rows are ordered according to the level of one of the variables presented.

Numerical precision

Spurious precision adds no value to a paper and even detracts from its readability and credibility. Results obtained from a calculator or computer usually need to be rounded. When presenting means, standard deviations, and other statistics the author should bear in mind the precision of the original data. Means should not normally be given to more than one decimal place more than the raw data, but standard deviations or standard errors may need to be quoted to one extra decimal place. It is rarely necessary to quote percentages to more than one decimal place, and even one decimal place is often not needed. With samples of less than 100 the use of decimal places implies unwarranted precision and should be avoided. Note that these remarks apply only to presentation of results—rounding should not be used before or during analysis. It is sufficient to quote values of t, χ^2 and r to two decimal places.

Miscellaneous technical terms

It is impossible to define here all statistical terms. The following comments relate to some terms which are frequently used in an incorrect or confusing manner.

Correlation should preferably not be used as a general term to describe any relationship. It has a specific technical meaning as a measure of association, for which it should be reserved in statistical work.

Incidence should be used to describe the rate of occurrence of new cases of a given characteristic in a study sample or population, such as the number of new notifications of cancer in one year. The proportion of a sample already having a characteristic is the prevalence.

Non-parametric refers to certain statistical analyses, such as the Mann–Whitney U test; it is not a characteristic of the observations themselves.

Parameter should not be used in place of "variable" to refer to a measurement or attribute on which observations are made. Parameters are characteristics of distributions or relationships in the population which are estimated by statistical analysis of a sample of observations.

Percentiles—When the range of values of a variable is divided into equal groups, the cut-off points are the median, tertiles, quartiles, quintiles, and so on; the groups themselves should be referred to as halves, thirds, quarters, fifths, etc.

Sensitivity is the ability of a test to identify a disease when it really is present—that is, the proportion positive of those who have the disease. *Specificity* is the ability of a test to identify the absence of a disease when the disease really is not present—that is, the proportion negative of those who do not have the disease. See also "Prediction and diagnostic tests", below.

Further guidance on terminology is given by Lang and Secic.[13]

Discussion section: interpretation

Interpretation of hypothesis tests

A hypothesis test assesses, by means of the probability P, the plausibility of the observed data when some "null hypothesis" (such as there being no difference between groups) is true. The P value is the probability that the observed data, or a more extreme outcome, would have occurred by chance—that is, just due to sampling variation—when the null hypothesis is true. If P is small one doubts the null hypothesis. If P is large the data are plausibly consistent with the null hypothesis, which thus cannot be rejected. P is not, therefore, the probability of there being no real effect.

Even if there is a large real effect a non-significant result is quite likely if the number of observations is small. Conversely, if the sample size is very large, a statistically significant result may occur when there is only a small real effect. Thus statistical significance should not be taken as synonymous with clinical importance.

The interpretation of the results of hypothesis tests largely follows from the above. A significant result does not necessarily indicate a real effect. There is always some risk of a false positive finding; this risk diminishes for smaller P values. Furthermore, a non-significant result (conventionally $P > 0.05$) does not mean that there is no effect but only that the data are compatible with there being no effect. Some flexibility is desirable in interpreting P values. The 0.05 level is a convenient cut-off point, but P values of 0.04 and 0.06, which are not greatly different, ought to lead to similar interpretations, rather than radically different ones. The designation of any result with $P > 0.05$ as not significant may thus mislead the reader (and the authors); hence the suggestion above ("Presentation of results of hypothesis tests") to quote actual P values.

Confidence intervals are extremely helpful in interpretation, particularly for small studies, as they show the degree of uncertainty related to a result—such as the difference between two means—whether or not it was statistically significant. Their use in conjunction with non-significant results may be especially enlightening.

Many hypothesis tests

In many research projects some tests of hypotheses relate to important comparisons that were envisaged when the research was initiated. Tests of hypotheses which were not decided in advance are subsidiary, especially if suggested by the results. It is important to distinguish these two cases and give much greater weight to the tests of those hypotheses that were formulated initially. Other tests should be considered as being only exploratory— for forming new hypotheses to be investigated in further studies. One reason for this is that when very many hypothesis tests are performed in the analysis of one study, perhaps comparing many subgroups or looking at many variables, a number of spurious positive results can be expected to arise by chance alone, which may pose considerable problems of interpretation. Clearly, the more tests that are carried out the greater is the likelihood of finding some significant results, but the expected number of false-positive findings will increase too. One way of allowing for the risk of false-positive results is to set a smaller level of P as a criterion of statistical significance.

A more complex problem arises when tests of significance are carried out on dependent (correlated) data. One example of this is in the analysis of serial data (discussed above—"Repeated measurements"), when the same test is performed on data for the same variable collected from the same subjects at different times. Another is where separate analyses of two or more correlated variables are carried out as if they were independent; any corroboration may not greatly increase the weight of evidence because the tests relate to similar data. For example, diastolic and systolic blood pressures behave very similarly, as may alternative ways of assessing patient response generally. Very careful interpretation of results is required in such cases.

Association and causality

A statistically significant association (obtained from correlation or χ^2 analysis) does not in itself provide direct evidence of a causal relationship between the variables concerned. In observational studies causality can be established only on non-statistical grounds; it is easier to infer causality in randomised trials. Great care should be taken in comparing variables which both vary with time, because it is easy to obtain apparent associations which are spurious.

Prediction and diagnostic tests

Even when regression analysis has indicated a statistically significant relationship between two variables, there may be considerable imprecision when using the regression equation to predict the numerical level of one variable (y) from the other (x) for individual cases. The accuracy of such predictions cannot be assessed from the correlation or regression coefficient but requires the calculation of the prediction interval for the estimated y value corresponding to a specific x value (see chapter 8). The regression line should be used only to predict the y variable from the x variable, and not the reverse.

A diagnostic test with a high sensitivity and specificity may not necessarily be a useful test for diagnostic purposes, especially when applied in a population where the prevalence of the disease is very low. It is useful here to calculate the proportion of subjects with positive test results who actually had the disease (known as the *positive predictive value*). Note that there is no consensus on the definition of "false-positive rate" or "false-negative rate"; it should always be made clear exactly what is being calculated, and this can best be illustrated by a 2×2 table relating the test results to the patients' true disease status.

A similar diagnostic problem arises with continuous variables. The classification as "abnormal" of values outside the "normal range" for a variable is common, but if the prevalence of true abnormality is low most values outside the normal range will be normal. The definition of abnormality should be based on both clinical and statistical criteria.

Weaknesses

It is better to address weaknesses in research design and execution, if one is aware of them, and to consider their possible effects on the results and their interpretation than to ignore them in the hope that they will not be noticed.

Concluding remarks

The purpose of statistical methods is to provide a straightforward factual account of the scientific evidence derived from a piece of research. The skills and experience needed to design suitable studies, carry out sensible statistical analyses, and communicate the findings in a clear and objective manner are not easy to acquire. While we hope that these guidelines help authors to avoid statistical pitfalls, we reiterate our earlier advice to seek the advice of a statistician when possible.

1 Altman DG. Statistics in medical journals. *Stat Med* 1982; **1**:59–71.
2 Andersen B. *Methodological errors in medical research.* Oxford, Blackwell Science, 1990.
3 Altman DG. The scandal of poor medical research. *BMJ* 1994;**308**:283–4.
4 O'Fallon JR, Dubey SB, Salsburg DS, *et al.* Should there be statistical guidelines for medical research papers? *Biometrics* 1978;**34**:687–95.
5 Bailar JC, Mosteller F. Guidelines for statistical reporting in articles for medical journals: amplifications and explanations. *Ann Intern Med* 1988;**108**:266–73.
6 International Committee of Medical Journal Editors. Uniform requirements for manuscripts submitted to biomedical journals. *JAMA* 1997;**277**:927–34.
7 Simon R, Wittes RE. Methodologic guidelines for reports of clinical trials. *Cancer Treat Rep* 1985;**69**:1–3.
8 Epidemiology Work Group of the Interagency Regulatory Liaison Group. Guidelines for the documentation of epidemiologic studies. *Am J Epidemiol* 1981;**114**:609–13.
9 Lichtenstein MJ, Mulrow CD, Elwood PC. Guidelines for reading case-control studies. *J Chron Dis* 1987;**40**:893–903.
10 Murray GD. Statistical guidelines for the *British Journal of Surgery*. *Br J Surgery* 1991;**78**:782–4.
11 Begg C, Cho M, Eastwood S, Horton R, Moher D, Olkin I, *et al.* Improving the quality of reporting of randomized controlled trials: the CONSORT statement. *JAMA* 1996;**276**:637–9.
12 Moher D, Cook DJ, Eastwood S, Olkin I, Rennie D, Stroup DF for the QUOROM group. Improving the quality of reports of meta-analyses of randomised controlled trials: the QUOROM statement. *Lancet* 1999;**354**:1896–900.

13 Lang TA and Secic M. *How to report statistics in medicine. Annotated guidelines for authors, editors, and reviewers.* Philadelphia: American College of Physicians, 1997.

14 Altman DG. *Practical statistics for medical research.* London: Chapman & Hall, 1991.

15 Armitage P, Berry G. *Statistical methods in medical research.* 3rd edn. Oxford: Blackwell Science, 1994.

16 Bland M. *An introduction to medical statistics.* 3rd edn. Oxford: Oxford University Press, 2000.

17 Campbell MJ, Machin D. *Medical statistics. A commonsense approach.* 3rd edn. Chichester: John Wiley, 1999.

18 Colton T. *Statistics in medicine.* Boston: Little, Brown, 1974.

19 Pocock SJ. *Clinical trials. A practical approach.* Chichester: John Wiley, 1983.

20 Altman DG. Randomisation. *BMJ* 1991;**302**:1481–2.

15 Statistical checklists

MARTIN J GARDNER, DAVID MACHIN,
MICHAEL J CAMPBELL,
DOUGLAS G ALTMAN

Introduction

The *British Medical Journal* (*BMJ*) uses two checklists to evaluate the statistical aspects of medical studies. These checklists were developed during statistical assessment of papers submitted to the journal.[1] One checklist is intended for all studies other than clinical trials and, because of this non-specific application, is limited in detail. The second is for controlled clinical trials and includes questions concerned with randomised comparisons of health interventions. Information on the principles behind the questions may be found in books[2,3] or in the statistical guidelines of chapter 14.

In addition to the two checklists that were developed to assist in the statistical evaluation of submitted manuscripts, it has been recognised that it is important that controlled trials are reported adequately. This has led to the development of the CONSORT guidelines for reporting.[4] The *BMJ* is one of over 70 journals which require authors to adhere to the CONSORT recommendations.

In this chapter, we discuss these three checklists in detail. At the end, we consider briefly checklists developed for some other types of study.

Uses of the checklists

The checklists may be used at different stages of manuscript assessment and study development.

Refereeing is difficult and time-consuming.[5-7] Submitted papers clearly require subject matter referees to judge their merit within the medical specialty. Most reports, however, have some statistical content that may be outside the expertise of these particular referees and warrant separate assessment. Many medical journals make extensive use of statisticians to assess medical papers.[8] Although the relevant considerations for this may be clear in a statistician's mind, a list of items to check and respond to serves as a useful reminder. These answers serve as the backbone for the statistician's recommendations on the paper and are supplemented by written comments.

Editorial staff find a checklist helpful in obtaining a summary view on a paper. Because of the fixed format they can develop a familiarity which allows more rapid evaluation than from a textual report. The latter will generally be needed as well, but will be shorter than a report without the checklist.

Authors receiving a copy of the completed checklist from the editor can see where their paper was thought to be statistically unsatisfactory, if that is the case. Suggestions for improvements will usually be given in the report if revision is suggested. Alternatively, problems with the design or conduct of the study making the paper unsuitable for publication will be pointed out; some examples are given by Vaisrub[9] and Altman.[7]

Planners of studies can be guided by the checklists, which indicate the need to consider relevant statistical aspects during development of protocols. Detailed advice may have to be sought from a statistician or in appropriate publications. Referral to the checklists should also improve the description of the statistical aspects of studies in submitted papers.

Outline of the *BMJ* checklists

General checklist

Aspects covered by the general checklist include design, conduct, analysis, and presentation of studies (Figure 15.1). For each question "yes" or "no" answers are sought, but in some cases "unclear" is allowed, though its use should be minimal.

The first part of the checklist relates to considerations before the start of an investigation, such as defining its main objective(s). Sometimes a choice of suitable studies to meet these is available, but some designs will be inappropriate. For example, it would not be sensible to compare elderly diseased patients with young healthy adults to determine whether a blood constituent is aetiologically important. Design considerations also include techniques

BMJ Ref No. _____ Date of review: _____

Design features

1	Is the objective of the study sufficiently described	Yes	Unclear	No
2	Was an appropriate study design used to achieve the objectives?	Yes	Unclear	No
3	Is there a satisfactory statement given of source of subjects?	Yes	Unclear	No
4	Is a pre-study calculation of required sample size reported?	Yes		No

Conduct of study

5	Was a satisfactory response rate achieved?	Yes	Unclear	No

Analysis and presentation

6	Is there a statement adequately describing or referencing all statistical procedures used?	Yes		No
7	Are the statistical analyses used appropriate?	Yes	Unclear	No
8	Is the presentation of statistical material satisfactory?	Yes		No
9	Are confidence intervals given for the main results?	Yes		No
10	Is the conclusion drawn from the statistical analysis justified?	Yes	Unclear	No

Recommendation on paper

11	Is the paper of acceptable statistical standard for publication?	Yes		No
12	If "No" to Question 11, could it become acceptable with suitable revision?	Yes		No

Reviewer:_____

Figure 15.1 Checklist for statistical review of general papers for the *BMJ*.

for measurement and collection of data. In addition, important statistical questions relate to the source and number of subjects studied. The former will be relevant to the validity of any generalised inferences from the results. The issue of the sample size required for a study is well documented, but many studies are still too small to detect anything other than large, and often unrealistic, effects.

When the study is under way, a high participation rate is needed from the recruited subjects. Those who do not participate fully are almost certain to be a biased group in some respects, with detrimental effects on the interpretation of the results. A comparison of relevant baseline characteristics of responders and non-responders should be given.[10]

The statistical methods used should be stated. If a technique is novel or unfamiliar then a description of its purpose and an outline of the method should be given together with a suitable reference. Aspects of presentation will also be checked, including tables and figures as well as textual content.

From the answers to the checklist, a summary can be made of the statistical content of a paper. Other features, which may be mentioned in the accompanying written report, contribute to the recommendation on its statistical quality.

Clinical trials checklist

For clinical trials, specific questions are asked in addition to the items from the general checklist (Figure 15.2).

At the design stage of a clinical trial, it is important to determine the diagnostic criteria for inclusion of subjects and to define clearly the treatments to be compared. Where a randomised study is appropriate, which usually is the case, a method of random allocation to treatment is mandatory and should be clearly described.[4,11] Unambiguous measures of outcome must be specified for trials comparing treatments and the duration of follow up stated. There are advantages if double-blind comparisons can be made, and treatment should start with a minimum delay after patient allocation. All these features should be described in the trial protocol.

In the Results section, the numbers and proportions of subjects treated and followed up should be stated. It is important also to describe dropouts and side effects by treatment group. In addition, treatment groups should be compared for relevant prognostic characteristics and adjustments for these made if appropriate in the analysis of outcome.

Comments on the *BMJ* checklists

These checklists have evolved over a period of time and, as shown in Figures 15.1 and 15.2, differ slightly from those used initially. For example, the question on confidence intervals (question 9 in the general checklist, question 23 in the clinical trials checklist) was added. It was included partly as a consequence of a change in *BMJ* policy.[12]

Statistical assessment is a possibility for any article submitted to the *BMJ*[13] and the checklists are used routinely in this. Such a statistical evaluation is one way to prevent the publication of papers with unsatisfactory statistical content. Other approaches are, of course, possible,[14] including the adoption of published statistical guidelines (such as in chapter 14) or having a statistician on the editorial board, or both. It should be recognised, though, that statistical errors remain common in medical journals despite the wide introduction of statistical refereeing.[8]

BMJ Ref No: _____ Date of Review: _____

Design features

		Yes	Unclear	No
1	Is the objective of the trial sufficiently described?	Yes	Unclear	No
2	Is there a satisfactory statement given of diagnostic criteria for entry to trial?	Yes	Unclear	No
3	Is there a satisfactory statement given of source of subjects?	Yes	Unclear	No
4	Were concurrent controls used (as opposed to historical controls)?	Yes	Unclear	No
5	Are the treatments well defined?	Yes	Unclear	No
6	Was random allocation to treatment used?	Yes	Unclear	No
7	Is the method of randomisation described?	Yes	Unclear	No
8	Was there an acceptably short delay from allocation to commencement of treatment?	Yes	Unclear	No
9	Was the potential degree of blindness used?	Yes	Unclear	No
10	Is there a satisfactory statement of criteria for outcome measures?	Yes	Unclear	No
11	Were the outcome measures appropriate?	Yes	Unclear	No
12	Is a pre-study calculation of required sample size reported?	Yes		No
13	Is the duration of post-treatment follow up stated?	Yes	Unclear	No

Conduct of trial

		Yes	Unclear	No
14	Are the treatment and control groups comparable in relevant measures?	Yes	Unclear	No
15	Were a high proportion of the subjects followed up?	Yes	Unclear	No
16	Did a high proportion of subjects complete treatment?	Yes	Unclear	No
17	Are the drop outs described by treatment/control groups?	Yes	Unclear	No
18	Are side effects of treatment reported?	Yes	Unclear	No

Analysis and presentation

		Yes	Unclear	No
19	Is there a statement adequately describing or referencing all statistical procedures used?	Yes		No
20	Are the statistical analyses used appropriate?	Yes	Unclear	No
21	Are prognostic factors adequately considered?	Yes	Unclear	No
22	Is the presentation of statistical material satisfactory?	Yes		No
23	Are confidence intervals given for the main results?	Yes		No
24	Is the conclusion drawn from the statistical analysis justified?	Yes	Unclear	No

Recommendation on paper

		Yes	No
25	Is the paper of acceptable statistical standard for publication?	Yes	No
26	If ''No'' to Question 25, could it become acceptable with suitable revision?	Yes	No

Reviewer: _____

Figure 15.2 Checklist for statistical review of papers on controlled clinical trials for the *BMJ*.

The checklists are intended for guidance on the statistical content of papers and are not presented as items to be covered at the expense of other important aspects of medical studies.[15,16]

Reporting randomised controlled trials: the CONSORT statement

It is widely recognised that randomised controlled trials are the best way to compare the effectiveness of different therapies. Only randomised trials allow one to make valid inferences of cause and effect. Randomised trials have considerable potential directly to affect patient care, occasionally as single trials, more often as the body of evidence from several trials, whether or not combined formally. It is thus entirely reasonable to require higher standards for papers reporting randomised trials than those describing other types of study.

Like all studies, randomised trials are open to bias if done badly.[17] It is thus essential that randomised trials are done well if they are to be reliable, but it is also important that they are reported adequately. Readers should not have to infer what was probably done—they should be told explicitly. Proper methodology should be used and be seen to have been used. Yet reviews of published trials have consistently found major deficiencies in reporting.[18–20] Those carrying out systematic reviews commonly find that the reporting of many randomised trials is poor, making their task much harder. Now, more than 50 years after the first publication of a randomised trial,[21] the guarantee of adequate reporting of these important studies is surely mandatory.

In 1994, two groups independently published proposals for requirements for the reporting of randomised trials.[22,23] A *JAMA* editorial suggested that the two groups should produce a unified statement.[24] The outcome was the CONSORT statement,[4] which includes a list of 21 items which should be reported in the paper (see Figure 15.3). There is also a flow chart describing patient progress through the trial, which should be included in the trial report (see Figure 15.4). In addition, a few specific subheadings are suggested within the Methods and Results sections of the paper. In the spirit of the times, the recommendations are evidence based where possible, with common sense dictating the remainder.

In essence, the requirement is that authors should provide enough information for readers to know how the trial was performed, so that they can judge whether the findings are likely to

Heading	Subheading	Descriptor	Reported? Yes or No
Title		1 Identify the study as a randomised trial.	_____
Abstract		2 Use a structured format.	_____
Introduction		3 State prospectively defined hypothesis, clinical objectives, and planned subgroup or covariate analyses.	_____
Methods	**Protocol**	**Describe**	
		4 Planned study population, together with inclusion and exclusion criteria.	_____
		5 Planned interventions and their timing.	_____
		6 Primary and secondary outcome measure(s) and the minimum important difference(s), and how the target sample size was projected.	_____
		7 Rationale and methods for statistical analyses, detailing main comparative analyses and whether they were completed on an intention-to-treat basis.	_____
		8 Prospectively defined stopping rules (if warranted).	_____
	Assignment	**Describe**	
		9 Unit of randomisation (e.g. individual, cluster, geographic).	_____
		10 Method used to generate the allocation schedule.	_____
		11 Method of allocation concealment and timing of assignment.	_____
		12 Method to separate the generator from the executor of assignment.	_____
	Masking	13 Describe mechanism (e.g. capsules, tablets); similarity of treatment characteristics (e.g. appearance, taste); allocation schedule control (location of code during trial and when broken); and evidence for successful masking (blinding) among participants, person doing intervention, outcome assessors, and data analysts.	_____
Results	**Participant flow and follow-up**	14 Provide a trial profile (see Figure 15.4) summarising participant flow, numbers and timing of randomisation assignment, interventions, and measurements for each randomised group.	_____
	Analysis	15 State estimated effect of intervention on primary and secondary outcome measures, including a point estimate and measure of precision (confidence interval).	_____
		16 State results in absolute numbers when feasible (e.g. 10/20 not 50%).	_____
		17 Present summary data and appropriate descriptive and inferential statistics in sufficient detail to permit alternative analyses and replication.	_____
		18 Describe prognostic variables by treatment group and any attempt to adjust for them.	_____
		19 Describe protocol deviations from the study as planned, together with the reasons.	_____
Comment		20 State specific interpretation of study findings, including sources of bias and imprecision (internal validity) and discussion of external validity, including appropriate quantitative measures when possible.	_____
		21 State general interpretation of the data in light of the totality of the available evidence.	_____

Figure 15.3 CONSORT checklist for randomised controlled trials.[4]

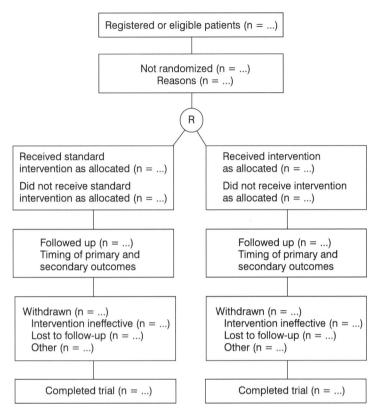

Figure 15.4 CONSORT patient flow diagram, showing progress through the various stages of a trial, including flow of participants, withdrawals, and timing of primary and secondary outcome measures. The "R" indicates randomisation.[4]

be reliable. The CONSORT suggestions mean that authors will no longer be able to hide study inadequacies by omission of important information. For example, authors can, and often do, hide their procedures behind the single word "randomised". Under CONSORT authors are required to give details of the randomisation. If authors have used an inferior approach, such as alternate allocation, they will have to say so. The *BMJ* has in fact refused to publish trials that were not truly randomised since 1991,[11] a position justified by subsequent empirical findings.[17,25]

As the authors note,[4] the checklist applies to the most common design—trials with two parallel groups. Some modification is needed for special types of trial, such as crossover trials and those with more than two treatment groups. Also, the list should be taken in addition to existing general requirements, for example to specify all statistical methods used in the analysis. This and other items appear on the checklist used by the *BMJ* referees which was discussed above.

Some of the items on the checklist would benefit from greater explanation than is possible in the CONSORT paper; in time, a fuller accompanying explanatory paper would be valuable. For example, while the advantages of randomisation have been apparent for several decades, understanding of the rationale for it remains poor and so its importance is not fully appreciated.[26]

The *BMJ* supports the CONSORT statement and has adopted the recommendations. So too have *JAMA, The Lancet,* and many other journals.[27] As a consequence, authors submitting reports of controlled trials to the *BMJ* should submit with their paper a copy of the completed checklist indicating on which page of the manuscript each item is addressed. The checklist is then used by the editors and the referees. The *BMJ* also use in the published papers the additional subheadings suggested by CONSORT.

It seems reasonable to hope that, in addition to improved reporting, the wide adoption of the CONSORT standard will improve the conduct of future trials by increasing awareness of the requirements for a good trial. Such success might lead to similar initiatives for other types of research.

Checklists for other types of study

While much methodological attention has focused on checklists for randomised controlled trials, some authors have produced checklists for assessing other types of study. Examples include epidemiological studies including case-control studies;[28,29] non-randomised studies;[30] evaluation of diagnostic and screening tests;[31,32] quality of life;[33] and economic evaluations.[34]

Finally, checklists and guidelines for the reporting of many methodological aspects of medical research matters are considered by Lang and Secic.[35]

1 Gardner MJ, Altman DG, Jones DR, Machin D. Is the statistical assessment of papers submitted to the "British Medical Journal" effective? *BMJ* 1983;**286**:1485–8.

2 Altman DG *Practical statistics for medical research*. London: Chapman and Hall, 1991.

3 Jadad AR. *Randomised controlled trials. A user's guide*. London: BMJ Books, 1998.

4 Begg C, Cho M, Eastwood S, Horton R, Moher D, Olkin I, *et al*. Improving the quality of reporting of randomized controlled trials: the CONSORT statement. *JAMA* 1996;**276**:637–9.

5 Lock S. *A difficult balance: editorial peer review in medicine*. London: Nuffield Provincial Hospitals Trust, 1985.

6 Godlee F, Jefferson T (eds). *Peer review in health sciences*. London: BMJ Books, 1999.

7 Altman DG. Statistical reviewing for medical journals. *Stat Med* 1998; **17**:2662–74.

8 Goodman SN, Altman DG, George SL. Statistical reviewing policies of medical journals—caveat lector? *J Gen Intern Med* 1998;**13**:753–6.

9 Vaisrub N. Manuscript review from a statistician's perspective. *JAMA* 1985; **253**:3145–7.

10 Evans SJW. Good surveys guide. *BMJ* 1991;**302**:302–3.

11 Altman DG. Randomisation. *BMJ* 1991;**302**:1481–2.

12 Langman MJS. Towards estimation and confidence intervals. *BMJ* 1986; **292**:716.

13 Advice to contributors. *BMJ* 1997;**314**:66–8 (also at http://www.bmj.com/).

14 George SL. Statistics in medical journals: a survey of current policies and proposals for editors. *Med Pediatr Oncol* 1985;**13**:109–12.

15 Jones RS. Statistical assessment of papers submitted to the "British Medical Journal". *BMJ* 1983;**286**:1971.

16 Healy MJR. Statistical guidelines for contributors to medical journals. *BMJ* 1983;**287**:132.

17 Schulz KF, Chalmers I, Hayes R, Altman DG. Empirical evidence of bias. Dimensions of methodological quality associated with estimates of treatment effects in controlled trials. *JAMA* 1995;**273**:408–12.

18 Mosteller F, Gilbert JP, McPeek B. Reporting standards and research strategies for controlled trials. Agenda for the editor. *Controlled Clin Trials* 1980;**1**:37–58.

19 Pocock SJ, Hughes MD, Lee RJ. Statistical problems in the reporting of clinical trials. *N Engl J Med* 1987;**317**:426–32.

20 Schulz KF, Chalmers I, Grimes DA, Altman DG. Assessing the quality of randomization from reports of controlled trials published in obstetrics and gynecology journals. *JAMA* 1994;**272**:125–8.

21 Medical Research Council. Streptomycin treatment of pulmonary tuberculosis. *BMJ* 1948;**ii**:769–82.

22 Standards of Reporting Trials Group. A proposal for structured reporting of randomized controlled trials. *JAMA* 1994;**272**:1926–31.

23 Working Group on Recommendations for Reporting of Clinical Trials in the Biomedical Literature. Call for comments on a proposal to improve reporting of clinical trials in the biomedical literature: a position paper. *Ann Intern Med* 1994;**121**:894–5.

24 Rennie D. Reporting randomized controlled trials: an experiment and a call for responses from readers. *JAMA* 1995;**273**:1054–5.

25 Moher D, Pham B, Jones A, Cook DJ, Jadad AR, Moher M, Tugwell P, Klassen TP. Does quality of reports of randomised trials affect estimates of intervention efficacy reported in meta-analyses? *Lancet* 1998;**352**:609–13.

26 Schulz KF. Subverting randomization in controlled trials. *JAMA* 1996; **274**:1456–8.

27 Moher D. CONSORT: An evolving tool to help improve the quality of reports of randomized controlled trials. *JAMA* 1998;**279**:1489–91.

28 Lichtenstein MJ, Mulrow CD, Elwood PC. Guidelines for reading case-control studies. *J Chron Dis* 1987;**40**:893–903.

29 Bracken MB. Reporting observational studies. *Br J Obstet Gynaecol* 1989; **96**:383–8.

30 Downs SH, Black N. The feasibility of creating a checklist for the assessment of the methodological quality both of randomised and non-randomised studies of health care interventions. *J Epidemiol Community Health* 1998;**52**:377–84.

31 Sheps SB, Schechter MT. The assessment of diagnostic tests. A survey of current medical research. *JAMA* 1984;**252**:2418–22.

32 Wald N, Cuckle H. Reporting the assessment of screening and diagnostic tests. *Br J Obstet Gynaecol* 1989;**96**:389–96.

33 Staquet MJ, Berzon RA, Osoba D, Machin D. Guidelines for reporting results of quality of life assessments in clinical trials. In Staquet MJ, Hays RD, Fayers PM (eds). *Quality of life assessment in clinical trials.* Oxford: Oxford University Press, 1998.

34 Drummond MF, Jefferson TO. Guidelines for authors and peer reviewers of economic submissions to the BMJ. *BMJ* 1996;**313**:275–83.

35 Lang TA and Secic M. *How to report statistics in medicine. Annotated guidelines for authors, editors, and reviewers.* Philadelphia: American College of Physicians, 1997.

Part III
Notation, software, and tables

16 Notation

DOUGLAS G ALTMAN

Chapters 4 to 1 1 contain formulae for calculating confidence intervals. Repeated use is made of the mathematical notation explained below.

$\bar{x}$ the mean of a sample of observations, where the individual observations are denoted by x or x_i; it is pronounced "x bar". In some chapters we use y and d to denote sets of observations and $\bar{y}$ and $\bar{d}$ to denote their means.

p the proportion with a certain characteristic in a sample of individuals.

SD (or s)   the standard deviation of a set of observations. It is a measure of their variability around the sample mean. s^2 is known as the variance.

SE   the standard error of the sample mean or some other estimated statistic. It is a measure of the uncertainty of such an estimate and is used to derive a confidence interval in most of the chapters in this book.

         (The distinct uses and interpretation of the SD and SE are discussed in appendix 1 of chapter 3. Note that the notation SE(b) means "the standard error of b.")

$\sum x$ the Greek capital letter sigma, denoting "sum of." Thus $\sum x$ means the sum of all the values of x. A more correct notation is $\sum_{i=1}^{n} x_i$, which means the sum of the n values of x_i; that is, $x_1 + x_2 + x_3 + \ldots + x_n$. The simpler notation $\sum x$ is used when it is clear which items are being added together.

$\prod x$ the Greek capital letter pi, denoting "product of." Thus $\prod x$ means the product of all the values of x. As with $\sum x$ above, a fuller notation is $\prod_{i=1}^{n} x_i$, which is equal to $x_1 \times x_2 \times x_3 \times \ldots \times x_n$, but the shorter notation is used when the meaning is clear (see chapter 9).

$(\ldots)$ brackets are used in formulae to clarify the structure and to indicate the correct method of calculation. The quantity inside brackets must always be calculated first. If there are brackets within brackets the inner quantity is evaluated first.

$\log_e x$ the logarithmic function giving the value y such that $x = e^y$, where e is the constant $2 \cdot 718\,281 \ldots$ $\log_e x$ is sometimes known as the natural logarithm of x, and an alternative notation is $\ln x$.

    A key feature of the logarithmic transformation is that it is often successful in converting a non-Normal skewed distribution into an approximately Normal distribution (see chapter 4). Calculations, such as those to derive a confidence interval, can be performed using the log data and the results back transformed using the function e^x (see next entry).

e^x the exponential function denoting the inverse procedure to taking natural logarithms. It is sometimes called an antilogarithmic transformation. An alternative notation is $\exp(x)$.

n or N the sample size.

n_i or N_i the sample size in the ith group of subjects.

$z_{1-\alpha/2}$; $z_{1-\alpha/2}$ represents a value from the "standard Normal
α;   distribution," which is the theoretical Normal distri-
$100(1-\alpha)$ bution with mean 0 and standard deviation 1 (see Figure 3.5). The subscript $1 - \alpha/2$ represents the proportion of the distribution below the value $z_{1-\alpha/2}$. Thus $z_{0 \cdot 975}$ is the value from the standard Normal distribution below which lies the bottom $0 \cdot 975$ (or $97 \cdot 5\%$) of the distribution. For this example, $\alpha = 0 \cdot 025$ (or $2 \cdot 5\%$).

    The central $1 - \alpha$, or $100(1 - \alpha)\%$, of the distribution lies between $z_{\alpha/2}$ and $z_{1-\alpha/2}$. Because of the symmetry of the Normal distribution $z_{\alpha/2} = -z_{1-\alpha/2}$, so that the central $100(1 - \alpha)\%$ of the distribution lies between $-z_{1-\alpha/2}$ and $z_{1-\alpha/2}$. For example, the central 0·95 (or 95%) of the Normal distribution lies between $-z_{0·975}$ and $z_{0·975}$; that is, between $-1·96$ and $+1·96$. See also appendix 2 of chapter 3.

(Note that in the first edition we used the notation $N_{1-\alpha/2}$ rather than $z_{1-\alpha/2}$.)

$t_{1-\alpha/2}$ For some estimates, such as means and regression coefficients, the distribution of values from repeated sampling has a t distribution rather than a Normal distribution. For large samples the t distribution becomes nearly the same as the Normal distribution, but for small samples it has longer tails. As the tails of the distribution are relevant when calculating a confidence interval it is important to use the t distribution when appropriate. The logic behind the notation $t_{1-\alpha/2}$, however, is exactly as for the Normal distribution described in the preceding entry.

The t distribution, and hence the value of $t_{1-\alpha/2}$, is different according to the size of the sample(s) of data and is characterised by the "degrees of freedom". The method for calculating the relevant degrees of freedom is given in those chapters which make use of the t distribution.

In many cases, both confidence intervals and hypothesis tests are calculated on the same data. It is important to remember that the value of the theoretical t distribution should be used for calculating a confidence interval, and not the observed value of the t statistic calculated in the hypothesis test.

P   the probability value (or significance level) obtained from a hypothesis test. P is the probability of the data (or some more extreme data) arising by chance—that is, due to sampling variation only—when the null hypothesis is true. Hypothesis testing is discussed in chapters 3, 13, and 14, but methods are not covered in detail in this book.

17 Computer software for calculating confidence intervals (CIA)

TREVOR N BRYANT

The first edition of *Statistics with confidence*[1] was complemented by the publication of the DOS program Confidence Interval Analysis (CIA).[2] The program has been rewritten completely for the Windows operating system and this new version accompanies this book. CIA now includes several new methods introduced in this second edition of the book, and also incorporates suggestions from users for the improvement of the original version.

This chapter describes the program in outline. The description is not intended to be an instruction manual; that task has been included in the help system that comes with CIA. For the technically minded, the software was developed using Borland Delphi v4.0 (Inprise Corporation) and ForHelp (ForeFront Technologies).

CIA provides confidence interval calculations as described in chapters 4 to 11 in this book. The sole purpose of CIA is to calculate confidence intervals. This can be done only at the 90%, 95%, or 99% level because these are the most widely reported values and we do not want to encourage the presentation of non-standard intervals. CIA has not been written as a general-purpose statistical package because there are already many good packages. However, their coverage of confidence intervals can be patchy and they may be presented in the results for one statistical procedure but not another.

Outline of the CIA program

CIA can either use raw data, which are entered via the Data Editor, or summary information, for example, cell totals, which are entered using the Method windows. The program displays three types of window:

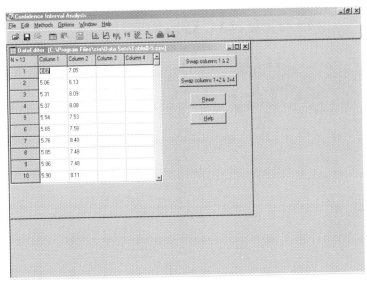

Figure 17.1 The Data Editor of CIA showing values read from a file created by exporting the data in CSV format from Excel.

The Data Editor window

Data can be entered into this window from the keyboard, copied and pasted from another application via the window's clipboard, for example from a spreadsheet, or read from a document such as a CSV (comma separated values) file created by Excel (see Figure 17.1). Data can be saved from the Data Editor to a document. Various checks are applied to the data as they are entered so that inappropriate values are trapped and excluded. The Data Editor is limited to 4000 rows of data, which should be sufficient to cope with most data sets.

The Method windows

The type of confidence interval required determines the chosen window which can be opened. The choice is made either by selecting Methods from the menu bar or by clicking on one of the method icons (see Figures 17.2 and 17.3). Each method has various tabbed options that depend on the statistical technique used. For example, with regression and correlation the confidence interval for the slope of a single line may be requested, or the confidence interval for the mean value of the outcome variable (y) may be needed (Figure 17.3). The summary statistics and the confidence interval calculation are

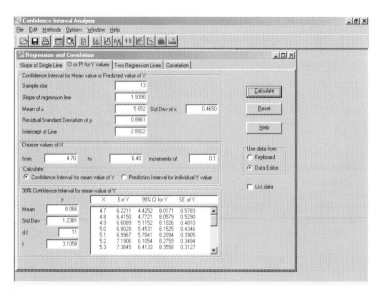

Figure 17.2 Calculation of a 95% confidence interval for the mean value of y for a regression line.

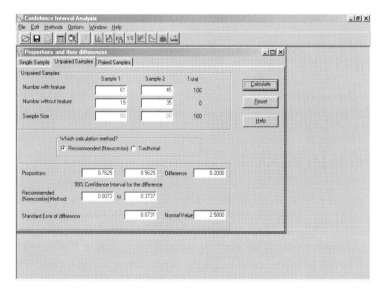

Figure 17.3 Calculation of a 99% confidence interval for the difference between two proportions.

displayed in the window. Where appropriate, warning messages are displayed. For example, a message may advise that the confidence interval calculation is inappropriate for the data provided.

A list of the confidence interval calculations performed by CIA is presented in Table 17.1. A few methods described in the book

Table 17.1 Confidence intervals calculated by CIA

Chapter		
4 Means and their differences	Single sample Two samples	Paired and unpaired data
5 Medians and their differences	Single sample Two samples	Paired and unpaired data
6 Proportions and their differences	Single sample Two samples	Paired and unpaired data
7 Epidemiological studies	Incidence study	
	Case-control study	Unmatched Series unmatched Matched
	Standardised ratios Ratio of two standardised ratios Standardised rates	
8 Regression and correlation	Single sample	Slope of the regression line Mean value of y for given value of x For the prediction of an individual value Correlation coefficient
	Two samples	Difference between slopes of two lines Common slope of two regression lines Vertical distance between two regression lines
9 Time to event studies	Single sample	Survival proportion Median survival time
	Two samples	Survival proportion Median survival time
	Hazard ratio	
10 Diagnostic studies	Sensitivity Specificity Positive and negative predictive value Likelihood ratio Area under ROC curve Kappa	
11 Clinical trials and meta-analyses	Number needed to treat Parallel group trials Crossover trials Crossover trial: relative risk	

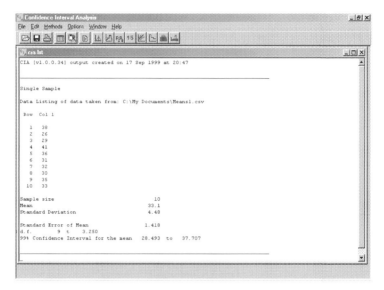

Figure 17.4 The Output window in CIA summarising the calculation of a 95% confidence interval for the mean.

are not included. These are mainly the more complex methods, such as those associated with multiple regression, for which standard statistical software should be used.

The Output window

A record of the calculations can be displayed in the output window (Figure 17.4). The contents of the output window can be printed or saved as a document. If this feature is not wanted it can be disabled.

Options in CIA

Apart from the use, or not, of the Output window, CIA allows the number of decimal places presented for the confidence intervals and associated statistics to be controlled. Three decimal places are given by default, although where summary statistics are calculated from raw data, these values are given to one (mean) or two (standard deviation) more decimal places than found in the data.

Confidence intervals can be calculated at the 90%, 95%, or 99% level. The value is set within the Options.

Options set by the user are stored between uses of CIA. The initial (default) settings can be reset.

Help

CIA comes with an extensive help system. Each window within the program has its own help link. Example data used in this book are provided as part of the help system and can be copied from the Help screen into the Data Editor.

Software updates and bug fixes

No matter how hard software authors try, the odd "bug" slips into all programs. We acknowledge that there may be bugs in CIA as no software is ever perfect. There is a website for CIA where updates to the software and bug fixes will be made available. The address is as follows: < www.medschool.soton.ac.uk/cia/main.htm > .

1 Gardner MJ, Altman DG (eds). *Statistics with confidence*. London: BMJ Publishing Group, 1989.
2 Gardner MJ, Gardner SB, Winter PD. *Confidence Interval Analysis (CIA)*. London: BMJ Publishing Group, 1989.

18 Tables for the calculation of confidence intervals

MARTIN J GARDNER

In each table selected values are given to enable the calculation of 90%, 95%, and 99% confidence intervals using the methods described in part I. For values applicable to other levels of confidence, reference should be made to more extensive published tables such as in *Geigy scientific tables*.[1] The first three tables can be used for calculating confidence intervals for a wide variety of statistics—such as means, proportions, regression analyses, and standardised mortality ratios—whereas the last three are for specific statistics, as described in chapter 5.

Table 18.1 Normal distribution
Table 18.2 *t* distribution
Table 18.3 Poisson distribution
Table 18.4 Median (single sample) or differences between medians (paired samples), based on Binomial distribution with probability $\frac{1}{2}$
Table 18.5 Differences between medians (unpaired samples), based on distributions of the Wilcoxon two sample rank sum test statistic and of the Mann–Whitney U test statistic
Table 18.6 Median (single sample) or differences between medians (paired samples), based on the distribution of the Wilcoxon matched pairs signed rank sum test statistic

The tables have been produced directly from theoretical formulae.

1 Lentner C, ed. *Geigy scientific tables*. Vol. 2. 8th ed. Basle: Ciba-Geigy, 1982.

Table 18.1 Values from the Normal distribution for use in calculating confidence intervals

The value tabulated is $z_{1-\alpha/2}$ from the standard Normal distribution for the $100(1 - \alpha/2)$ percentile and is to be used in finding $100(1 - \alpha)\%$ confidence intervals. For a 90% confidence interval α is 0·10, for a 95% confidence interval α is 0·05, and for a 99% confidence interval α is 0·01.

Level of confidence		
90%	95%	99%
1·645	1·960	2·576

Table 18.2 Values from the *t* distribution for 1 to 400 degrees of freedom for use in calculating confidence intervals

The value tabulated is $t_{1-\alpha/2}$ from the t distribution for the $100(1-\alpha/2)$ percentile and is to be used in finding $100(1-\alpha)\%$ confidence intervals. For a 90% confidence interval α is 0·10, for a 95% confidence interval α is 0·05, and for a 99% confidence interval α is 0·01. The relation of the degrees of freedom to sample size(s) depends on the particular application and is described in chapters 3, 4, and 8 where appropriate.

Degrees of freedom	Level of confidence			Degrees of freedom	Level of confidence		
	90%	95%	99%		90%	95%	99%
1	6·314	12·706	63·657	44	1·680	2·015	2·692
2	2·920	4·303	9·925	45	1·679	2·014	2·690
3	2·353	3·182	5·841	46	1·679	2·013	2·687
4	2·132	2·776	4·604	47	1·678	2·012	2·685
5	2·015	2·571	4·032	48	1·677	2·011	2·682
6	1·943	2·447	3·707	49	1·677	2·010	2·680
7	1·895	2·365	3·499	50	1·676	2·009	2·678
8	1·860	2·306	3·355	51	1·675	2·008	2·676
9	1·833	2·262	3·250	52	1·675	2·007	2·674
10	1·812	2·228	3·169	53	1·674	2·006	2·672
11	1·796	2·201	3·106	54	1·674	2·005	2·670
12	1·782	2·179	3·055	55	1·673	2·004	2·668
13	1·771	2·160	3·012	56	1·673	2·003	2·667
14	1·761	2·145	2·977	57	1·672	2·002	2·665
15	1·753	2·131	2·947	58	1·672	2·002	2·663
16	1·746	2·120	2·921	59	1·671	2·001	2·662
17	1·740	2·110	2·898	60	1·671	2·000	2·660
18	1·734	2·101	2·878	61	1·670	2·000	2·659
19	1·729	2·093	2·861	62	1·670	1·999	2·657
20	1·725	2·086	2·845	63	1·669	1·998	2·656
21	1·721	2·080	2·831	64	1·669	1·998	2·655
22	1·717	2·074	2·819	65	1·669	1·997	2·654
23	1·714	2·069	2·807	66	1·668	1·997	2·652
24	1·711	2·064	2·797	67	1·668	1·996	2·651
25	1·708	2·060	2·787	68	1·668	1·995	2·650
26	1·706	2·056	2·779	69	1·667	1·995	2·649
27	1·703	2·052	2·771	70	1·667	1·994	2·648
28	1·701	2·048	2·763	71	1·667	1·994	2·647
29	1·699	2·045	2·756	72	1·666	1·993	2·646
30	1·697	2·042	2·750	73	1·666	1·993	2·645
31	1·696	2·040	2·744	74	1·666	1·993	2·644
32	1·694	2·037	2·738	75	1·665	1·992	2·643
33	1·692	2·035	2·733	76	1·665	1·992	2·642
34	1·691	2·032	2·728	77	1·665	1·991	2·641
35	1·690	2·030	2·724	78	1·665	1·991	2·640
36	1·688	2·028	2·719	79	1·664	1·990	2·640
37	1·687	2·026	2·715	80	1·664	1·990	2·639
38	1·686	2·024	2·712	81	1·664	1·990	2·638
39	1·685	2·023	2·708	82	1·664	1·989	2·637
40	1·684	2·021	2·704	83	1·663	1·989	2·636
41	1·683	2·020	2·701	84	1·663	1·989	2·636
42	1·682	2·018	2·698	85	1·663	1·988	2·635
43	1·681	2·017	2·695	86	1·663	1·988	2·634

Table 18.2 (*continued*)

Degrees of freedom	Level of confidence			Degrees of freedom	Level of confidence		
	90%	95%	99%		90%	95%	99%
87	1·663	1·988	2·634	137	1·656	1·977	2·612
88	1·662	1·987	2·633	138	1·656	1·977	2·612
89	1·662	1·987	2·632	139	1·656	1·977	2·612
90	1·662	1·987	2·632	140	1·656	1·977	2·611
91	1·662	1·986	2·631	141	1·656	1·977	2·611
92	1·662	1·986	2·630	142	1·656	1·977	2·611
93	1·661	1·986	2·630	143	1·656	1·977	2·611
94	1·661	1·986	2·629	144	1·656	1·977	2·610
95	1·661	1·985	2·629	145	1·655	1·976	2·610
96	1·661	1·985	2·628	146	1·655	1·976	2·610
97	1·661	1·985	2·627	147	1·655	1·976	2·610
98	1·661	1·984	2·627	148	1·655	1·976	2·609
99	1·660	1·984	2·626	149	1·655	1·976	2·609
100	1·660	1·984	2·626	150	1·655	1·976	2·609
101	1·660	1·984	2·625	151	1·655	1·976	2·609
102	1·660	1·983	2·625	152	1·655	1·976	2·609
103	1·660	1·983	2·624	153	1·655	1·976	2·608
104	1·660	1·983	2·624	154	1·655	1·975	2·608
105	1·660	1·983	2·623	155	1·655	1·975	2·608
106	1·659	1·983	2·623	156	1·655	1·975	2·608
107	1·659	1·982	2·623	157	1·655	1·975	2·608
108	1·659	1·982	2·622	158	1·655	1·975	2·607
109	1·659	1·982	2·622	159	1·654	1·975	2·607
110	1·659	1·982	2·621	160	1·654	1·975	2·607
111	1·659	1·982	2·621	161	1·654	1·975	2·607
112	1·659	1·981	2·620	162	1·654	1·975	2·607
113	1·658	1·981	2·620	163	1·654	1·975	2·606
114	1·658	1·981	2·620	164	1·654	1·975	2·606
115	1·658	1·981	2·619	165	1·654	1·974	2·606
116	1·658	1·981	2·619	166	1·654	1·974	2·606
117	1·658	1·980	2·619	167	1·654	1·974	2·606
118	1·658	1·980	2·618	168	1·654	1·974	2·605
119	1·658	1·980	2·618	169	1·654	1·974	2·605
120	1·658	1·980	2·617	170	1·654	1·974	2·605
121	1·658	1·980	2·617	171	1·654	1·974	2·605
122	1·657	1·980	2·617	172	1·654	1·974	2·605
123	1·657	1·979	2·616	173	1·654	1·974	2·605
124	1·657	1·979	2·616	174	1·654	1·974	2·604
125	1·657	1·979	2·616	175	1·654	1·974	2·604
126	1·657	1·979	2·615	176	1·654	1·974	2·604
127	1·657	1·979	2·615	177	1·654	1·973	2·604
128	1·657	1·979	2·615	178	1·653	1·973	2·604
129	1·657	1·979	2·614	179	1·653	1·973	2·604
130	1·657	1·978	2·614	180	1·653	1·973	2·603
131	1·657	1·978	2·614	181	1·653	1·973	2·603
132	1·656	1·978	2·614	182	1·653	1·973	2·603
133	1·656	1·978	2·613	183	1·653	1·973	2·603
134	1·656	1·978	2·613	184	1·653	1·973	2·603
135	1·656	1·978	2·613	185	1·653	1·973	2·603
136	1·656	1·978	2·612	186	1·653	1·973	2·603

Table 18.2 (*continued*)

Degrees of freedom	Level of confidence			Degrees of freedom	Level of confidence		
	90%	95%	99%		90%	95%	99%
187	1·653	1·973	2·602	250	1·651	1·969	2·596
188	1·653	1·973	2·602	260	1·651	1·969	2·595
189	1·653	1·973	2·602	270	1·651	1·969	2·594
190	1·653	1·973	2·602	280	1·650	1·968	2·594
191	1·653	1·972	2·602	290	1·650	1·968	2·593
192	1·653	1·972	2·602	300	1·650	1·968	2·592
193	1·653	1·972	2·602	310	1·650	1·968	2·592
194	1·653	1·972	2·601	320	1·650	1·967	2·591
195	1·653	1·972	2·601	330	1·649	1·967	2·591
196	1·653	1·972	2·601	340	1·649	1·967	2·590
197	1·653	1·972	2·601	350	1·649	1·967	2·590
198	1·653	1·972	2·601	360	1·649	1·967	2·590
199	1·653	1·972	2·601	370	1·649	1·966	2·589
200	1·653	1·972	2·601	380	1·649	1·966	2·589
210	1·652	1·971	2·599	390	1·649	1·966	2·588
220	1·652	1·971	2·598	400	1·649	1·966	2·588
230	1·652	1·970	2·597	∞	1·645	1·960	2·576
240	1·651	1·970	2·596				

Table 18.3 Values from the Poisson distribution for observed numbers of from 0 to 100 for use in calculating confidence intervals

If x is the observed number in the study then the values tabulated (x_L to x_U) give the 100(1 − α)% confidence interval for the population mean, assuming that the observed number is from a Poisson distribution. For a 90% confidence interval α is 0·10, for a 95% confidence interval α is 0·05, and for a 99% confidence interval α is 0·01.

	Level of confidence					
	90%		95%		99%	
x	x_L	x_U	x_L	x_U	x_L	x_U
0	0	2·996	0	3·689	0	5·298
1	0·051	4·744	0·025	5·572	0·005	7·430
2	0·355	6·296	0·242	7·225	0·103	9·274
3	0·818	7·754	0·619	8·767	0·338	10·977
4	1·366	9·154	1·090	10·242	0·672	12·594
5	1·970	10·513	1·623	11·668	1·078	14·150
6	2·613	11·842	2·202	13·059	1·537	15·660
7	3·285	13·148	2·814	14·423	2·037	17·134
8	3·981	14·435	3·454	15·763	2·571	18·578
9	4·695	15·705	4·115	17·085	3·132	19·998
10	5·425	16·962	4·795	18·390	3·717	21·398
11	6·169	18·208	5·491	19·682	4·321	22·779
12	6·924	19·443	6·201	20·962	4·943	24·145
13	7·690	20·669	6·922	22·230	5·580	25·497
14	8·464	21·886	7·654	23·490	6·231	26·836
15	9·246	23·097	8·395	24·740	6·893	28·164
16	10·036	24·301	9·145	25·983	7·567	29·482
17	10·832	25·499	9·903	27·219	8·251	30·791
18	11·634	26·692	10·668	28·448	8·943	32·091
19	12·442	27·879	11·439	29·671	9·644	33·383
20	13·255	29·062	12·217	30·888	10·353	34·668
21	14·072	30·240	12·999	32·101	11·069	35·946
22	14·894	31·415	13·787	33·308	11·792	37·218
23	15·719	32·585	14·580	34·511	12·521	38·484
24	16·549	33·752	15·377	35·710	13·255	39·745
25	17·382	34·916	16·179	36·905	13·995	41·000
26	18·219	36·077	16·984	38·096	14·741	42·251
27	19·058	37·234	17·793	39·284	15·491	43·497
28	19·901	38·389	18·606	40·468	16·245	44·738
29	20·746	39·541	19·422	41·649	17·004	45·976
30	21·594	40·691	20·241	42·827	17·767	47·209
31	22·445	41·838	21·063	44·002	18·534	48·439
32	23·297	42·982	21·888	45·174	19·305	49·665
33	24·153	44·125	22·716	46·344	20·079	50·888
34	25·010	45·266	23·546	47·512	20·857	52·107
35	25·870	46·404	24·379	48·677	21·638	53·324
36	26·731	47·541	25·214	49·839	22·422	54·537
37	27·595	48·675	26·051	51·000	23·208	55·748
38	28·460	49·808	26·891	52·158	23·998	56·955
39	29·327	50·940	27·733	53·314	24·791	58·161
40	30·196	52·069	28·577	54·469	25·586	59·363
41	31·066	53·197	29·422	55·621	26·384	60·563

Table 18.3 (*continued*)

	Level of confidence						
	90%			95%		99%	
x	x_L	x_U		x_L	x_U	x_L	x_U
42	31·938	54·324		30·270	56·772	27·184	61·761
43	32·812	55·449		31·119	57·921	27·986	62·956
44	33·687	56·573		31·970	59·068	28·791	64·149
45	34·563	57·695		32·823	60·214	29·598	65·341
46	35·441	58·816		33·678	61·358	30·407	66·530
47	36·320	59·935		34·534	62·500	31·218	67·717
48	37·200	61·054		35·391	63·641	32·032	68·902
49	38·082	62·171		36·250	64·781	32·847	70·085
50	38·965	63·287		37·111	65·919	33·664	71·266
51	39·849	64·402		37·973	67·056	34·483	72·446
52	40·734	65·516		38·836	68·191	35·303	73·624
53	41·620	66·628		39·701	69·325	36·125	74·800
54	42·507	67·740		40·566	70·458	36·949	75·974
55	43·396	68·851		41·434	71·590	37·775	77·147
56	44·285	69·960		42·302	72·721	38·602	78·319
57	45·176	71·069		43·171	73·850	39·431	79·489
58	46·067	72·177		44·042	74·978	40·261	80·657
59	46·959	73·284		44·914	76·106	41·093	81·824
60	47·852	74·390		45·786	77·232	41·926	82·990
61	48·746	75·495		46·660	78·357	42·760	84·154
62	49·641	76·599		47·535	79·481	43·596	85·317
63	50·537	77·702		48·411	80·604	44·433	86·479
64	51·434	78·805		49·288	81·727	45·272	87·639
65	52·331	79·907		50·166	82·848	46·111	88·798
66	53·229	81·008		51·044	83·968	46·952	89·956
67	54·128	82·108		51·924	85·088	47·794	91·112
68	55·028	83·208		52·805	86·206	48·637	92·269
69	55·928	84·306		53·686	87·324	49·482	93·423
70	56·830	85·405		54·568	88·441	50·327	94·577
71	57·732	86·502		55·452	89·557	51·174	95·729
72	58·634	87·599		56·336	90·672	52·022	96·881
73	59·537	88·695		57·220	91·787	52·871	98·031
74	60·441	89·790		58·106	92·900	53·720	99·180
75	61·346	90·885		58·992	94·013	54·571	100·328
76	62·251	91·979		59·879	95·125	55·423	101·476
77	63·157	93·073		60·767	96·237	56·276	102·622
78	64·063	94·166		61·656	97·348	57·129	103·767
79	64·970	95·258		62·545	98·458	57·984	104·912
80	65·878	96·350		63·435	99·567	58·840	106·056
81	66·786	97·441		64·326	100·676	59·696	107·198
82	67·965	98·532		65·217	101·784	60·553	108·340
83	68·604	99·622		66·109	102·891	61·412	109·481
84	69·514	100·712		67·002	103·998	62·271	110·621
85	70·425	101·801		67·895	105·104	63·131	111·761
86	71·336	102·889		68·789	106·209	63·991	112·899
87	72·247	103·977		69·683	107·314	64·853	114·037
88	73·159	105·065		70·579	108·418	65·715	115·174
89	74·071	106·152		71·474	109·522	66·578	116·310

Table 18.3 (*continued*)

	Level of confidence					
	90%		95%		99%	
x	x_L	x_U	x_L	x_U	x_L	x_U
90	74·984	107·239	72·371	110·625	67·442	117·445
91	75·898	108·325	73·268	111·728	68·307	118·580
92	76·812	109·410	74·165	112·830	69·172	119·714
93	77·726	110·495	75·063	113·931	70·038	120·847
94	78·641	111·580	75·962	115·032	70·905	121·980
95	79·556	112·664	76·861	116·133	71·773	123·112
96	80·472	113·748	77·760	117·232	72·641	124·243
97	81·388	114·832	78·660	118·332	73·510	125·373
98	82·305	115·915	79·561	119·431	74·379	126·503
99	83·222	116·997	80·462	120·529	75·250	127·632
100	84·139	118·079	81·364	121·627	76·120	128·761

For $x > 100$ the following calculations can be carried out to obtain approximate values for x_L and x_U:

$$x_L = \left(\frac{z_{1-\alpha/2}}{2} - \sqrt{x} \right)^2 \quad \text{and} \quad x_U = \left(\frac{z_{1-\alpha/2}}{2} + \sqrt{x+1} \right)^2,$$

where $z_{1-\alpha/2}$ is the appropriate value from the standard Normal distribution for the $100(1 - \alpha/2)$ percentile.

As an example of the closeness of the approximations to the exact values, for $\alpha = 0.05$ ($z_{1-\alpha/2} = 1.96$) and $x = 100$ the formulae give $x_L = 81·360$ and $x_U = 121·658$ for the 95% confidence interval compared to the values of $x_L = 81·364$ and $x_U = 121·627$ tabulated above.

Table 18.4 Ranks of the observations for use in calculating confidence intervals for population medians in single samples or for differences between population medians for the case of two paired samples with sample sizes from 6 to 100 and the associated exact levels of confidence, based on the Binomial distribution with probability $\frac{1}{2}$.

The values tabulated (r_L to r_U) show the ranks of the observations to be used to give the approximate $100(1 - \alpha)\%$ confidence interval for the population median. For a 90% confidence interval α is 0·10, for a 95% confidence interval α is 0·05, and for a 99% confidence internal α is 0·01.

Sample size (n)	Level of confidence								
	90% (approx)			95% (approx)			99% (approx)		
	r_L	r_U	Exact level (%)	r_L	r_U	Exact level (%)	r_L	r_U	Exact level (%)
6	1	6	96·9	1	6	96·9	—	—	—
7	1	7	98·4	1	7	98·4	—	—	—
8	2	7	93·0	1	8	99·2	1	8	99·2
9	2	8	96·1	2	8	96·1	1	9	99·6
10	2	9	97·9	2	9	97·9	1	10	99·8
11	3	9	93·5	2	10	98·8	1	11	99·9
12	3	10	96·1	3	10	96·1	2	11	99·4
13	4	10	90·8	3	11	97·8	2	12	99·7
14	4	11	94·3	3	12	98·7	2	13	99·8
15	4	12	96·5	4	12	96·5	3	13	99·3
16	5	12	92·3	4	13	97·9	3	14	99·6
17	5	13	95·1	5	13	95·1	3	15	99·8
18	6	13	90·4	5	14	96·9	4	15	99·2
19	6	14	93·6	5	15	98·1	4	16	99·6
20	6	15	95·9	6	15	95·9	4	17	99·7
21	7	15	92·2	6	16	97·3	5	17	99·3
22	7	16	94·8	6	17	98·3	5	18	99·6
23	8	16	90·7	7	17	96·5	5	19	99·7
24	8	17	93·6	7	18	97·7	6	19	99·3
25	8	18	95·7	8	18	95·7	6	20	99·6
26	9	18	92·4	8	19	97·1	7	20	99·1
27	9	19	94·8	8	20	98·1	7	21	99·4
28	10	19	91·3	9	20	96·4	7	22	99·6
29	10	20	93·9	9	21	97·6	8	22	99·2
30	11	20	90·1	10	21	95·7	8	23	99·5
31	11	21	92·9	10	22	97·1	8	24	99·7
32	11	22	95·0	10	23	98·0	9	24	99·3
33	12	22	92·0	11	23	96·5	9	25	99·5
34	12	23	94·2	11	24	97·6	10	25	99·1
35	13	23	91·0	12	24	95·9	10	26	99·4
36	13	24	93·5	12	25	97·1	10	27	99·6
37	14	24	90·1	13	25	95·3	11	27	99·2
38	14	25	92·7	13	26	96·6	11	28	99·5
39	14	26	94·7	13	27	97·6	12	28	99·1
40	15	26	91·9	14	27	96·2	12	29	99·4
41	15	27	94·0	14	28	97·2	12	30	99·6
42	16	27	91·2	15	28	95·6	13	30	99·2
43	16	28	93·4	15	29	96·8	13	31	99·5

Table 18.4 (*continued*)

Sample size (*n*)	90% (approx)			95% (approx)			99% (approx)		
	r_L	r_U	Exact level (%)	r_L	r_U	Exact level (%)	r_L	r_U	Exact level (%)
44	17	28	90·4	16	29	95·1	14	31	99·0
45	17	29	92·8	16	30	96·4	14	32	99·3
46	17	30	94·6	16	31	97·4	14	33	99·5
47	18	30	92·1	17	31	96·0	15	33	99·2
48	18	31	94·1	17	32	97·1	15	34	99·4
49	19	31	91·5	18	32	95·6	16	34	99·1
50	19	32	93·5	18	33	96·7	16	35	99·3
51	20	32	90·8	19	33	95·1	16	36	99·5
52	20	33	93·0	19	34	96·4	17	36	99·2
53	21	33	90·2	19	35	97·3	17	37	99·5
54	21	34	92·4	20	35	96·0	18	37	99·1
55	21	35	94·2	20	36	97·0	18	38	99·4
56	22	35	91·9	21	36	95·6	18	39	99·5
57	22	36	93·7	21	37	96·7	19	39	99·2
58	23	36	91·3	22	37	95·2	19	40	99·5
59	23	37	93·3	22	38	96·4	20	40	99·1
60	24	37	90·8	22	39	97·3	20	41	99·4
61	24	38	92·8	23	39	96·0	21	41	99·0
62	25	38	90·2	23	40	97·0	21	42	99·3
63	25	39	92·3	24	40	95·7	21	43	99·5
64	25	40	94·0	24	41	96·7	22	43	99·2
65	26	40	91·8	25	41	95·4	22	44	99·4
66	26	41	93·6	25	42	96·4	23	44	99·1
67	27	41	91·4	26	42	95·0	23	45	99·3
68	27	42	93·2	26	43	96·2	23	46	99·5
69	28	42	90·9	26	44	97·1	24	46	99·2
70	28	43	92·8	27	44	95·9	24	47	99·4
71	29	43	90·4	27	45	96·8	25	47	99·1
72	29	44	92·4	28	45	95·6	25	48	99·4
73	29	45	94·0	28	46	96·6	26	48	99·0
74	30	45	91·9	29	46	95·3	26	49	99·3
75	30	46	93·6	29	47	96·3	26	50	99·5
76	31	46	91·5	29	48	97·1	27	50	99·2
77	31	47	93·2	30	48	96·0	27	51	99·4
78	32	47	91·1	30	49	96·9	28	51	99·1
79	32	48	92·9	31	49	95·8	28	52	99·3
80	33	48	90·7	31	50	96·7	29	52	99·0
81	33	49	92·5	32	50	95·5	29	53	99·3
82	34	49	90·3	32	51	96·5	29	54	99·5
83	34	50	92·2	33	51	95·2	30	54	99·2
84	34	51	93·7	33	52	96·2	30	55	99·4
85	35	51	91·8	33	53	97·1	31	55	99·1
86	35	52	93·4	34	53	96·0	31	56	99·3
87	36	52	91·4	34	54	96·9	32	56	99·0
88	36	53	93·1	35	54	95·8	32	57	99·3
89	37	53	91·1	35	55	96·7	32	58	99·4
90	37	54	92·8	36	55	95·5	33	58	99·2

Table 18.4 (*continued*)

Sample size (n)	90% (approx)			95% (approx)			99% (approx)		
	r_L	r_U	Exact level (%)	r_L	r_U	Exact level (%)	r_L	r_U	Exact level (%)
91	38	54	90·7	36	56	96·5	33	59	99·4
92	38	55	92·4	37	56	95·3	34	59	99·1
93	39	55	90·3	37	57	96·2	34	60	99·3
94	39	56	92·1	38	57	95·1	35	60	99·0
95	39	57	93·6	38	58	96·0	35	61	99·3
96	40	57	91·8	38	59	96·8	35	62	99·4
97	40	58	93·3	39	59	95·8	36	62	99·2
98	41	58	91·5	39	60	96·7	36	63	99·4
99	41	59	93·0	40	60	95·6	37	63	99·1
100	42	59	91·1	40	61	96·5	37	64	99·3

For sample sizes of n over 100, satisfactory approximations to the values of r_L and r_U can be found as described in chapter 5.

For $n = 100$ and $\alpha = 0.01$, for example, the calculations give $r = 37.1$ and $s = 63.9$, which rounded to the nearest integer give $r_L = 37$ and $r_U = 64$ for finding the 99% confidence interval, the same values as shown in the table.

For an explanation of the use of this table see chapter 5.

Table 18.5 Values of K for use in calculating confidence intervals for differences between population medians for the case of two unpaired samples with sample sizes n_1 and n_2 from 5 to 25 and the associated exact levels of confidence, based on the Wilcoxon two sample rank sum distribution

Sample sizes (n_1, n_2)		Level of confidence					
		90% (approx)		95% (approx)		99% (approx)	
Smaller	Larger	K	Exact level (%)	K	Exact level (%)	K	Exact level (%)
5	5	5	90·5	3	96·8	1	99·2
5	6	6	91·8	4	97·0	2	99·1
5	7	7	92·7	6	95·2	2	99·5
5	8	9	90·7	7	95·5	3	99·4
5	9	10	91·7	8	95·8	4	99·3
5	10	12	90·1	9	96·0	5	99·2
5	11	13	91·0	10	96·2	6	99·1
5	12	14	91·8	12	95·2	7	99·1
5	13	16	90·5	13	95·4	8	99·0
5	14	17	91·3	14	95·6	8	99·3
5	15	19	90·2	15	95·8	9	99·2
5	16	20	90·9	16	96·0	10	99·2
5	17	21	91·5	18	95·2	11	99·1
5	18	23	90·6	19	95·4	12	99·1
5	19	24	91·2	20	95·6	13	99·1
5	20	26	90·3	21	95·8	14	99·0
5	21	27	90·9	23	95·1	15	99·0
5	22	29	90·1	24	95·3	15	99·2
5	23	30	90·6	25	95·5	16	99·2
5	24	31	91·1	26	95·6	17	99·1
5	25	33	90·4	28	95·1	18	99·1
6	6	8	90·7	6	95·9	3	99·1
6	7	9	92·7	7	96·5	4	99·2
6	8	11	91·9	9	95·7	5	99·2
6	9	13	91·2	11	95·0	6	99·2
6	10	15	90·7	12	95·8	7	99·3
6	11	17	90·2	14	95·2	8	99·3
6	12	18	91·7	15	95·9	10	99·0
6	13	20	91·3	17	95·4	11	99·1
6	14	22	90·9	18	95·9	12	99·1
6	15	24	90·5	20	95·5	13	99·2
6	16	26	90·2	22	95·1	14	99·2
6	17	27	91·4	23	95·6	16	99·0
6	18	29	91·0	25	95·3	17	99·1
6	19	31	90·8	26	95·7	18	99·1
6	20	33	90·5	28	95·4	19	99·1
6	21	35	90·3	30	95·1	20	99·2
6	22	37	90·0	31	95·5	22	99·0
6	23	38	91·0	33	95·3	23	99·1
6	24	40	90·7	34	95·6	24	99·1
6	25	42	90·5	36	95·4	25	99·1

Table 18.5 (*continued*)

Sample sizes (n_1, n_2)		90% (approx)		95% (approx)		99% (approx)	
				Level of confidence			
Smaller	Larger	K	Exact level (%)	K	Exact level (%)	K	Exact level (%)
7	7	12	90·3	9	96·2	5	99·3
7	8	14	90·6	11	96·0	7	99·1
7	9	16	90·9	13	95·8	8	99·2
7	10	18	91·2	15	95·7	10	99·0
7	11	20	91·5	17	95·6	11	99·2
7	12	22	91·7	19	95·5	13	99·0
7	13	25	90·3	21	95·4	14	99·2
7	14	27	90·6	23	95·4	16	99·0
7	15	29	90·9	25	95·3	17	99·1
7	16	31	91·1	27	95·3	19	99·0
7	17	34	90·1	29	95·3	20	99·1
7	18	36	90·3	31	95·3	22	99·1
7	19	38	90·6	33	95·2	23	99·2
7	20	40	90·8	35	95·2	25	99·1
7	21	42	91·0	37	95·2	26	99·2
7	22	45	90·2	39	95·2	28	99·1
7	23	47	90·4	41	95·2	30	99·0
7	24	49	90·6	43	95·2	31	99·1
7	25	51	90·8	45	95·2	33	99·0
8	8	16	91·7	14	95·0	8	99·3
8	9	19	90·7	16	95·4	10	99·2
8	10	21	91·7	18	95·7	12	99·1
8	11	24	90·9	20	95·9	14	99·1
8	12	27	90·2	23	95·3	16	99·0
8	13	29	91·1	25	95·5	18	99·0
8	14	32	90·5	27	95·8	19	99·2
8	15	34	91·3	30	95·3	21	99·2
8	16	37	90·7	32	95·5	23	99·1
8	17	40	90·3	35	95·1	25	99·1
8	18	42	91·0	37	95·3	27	99·1
8	19	45	90·5	39	95·5	29	99·1
8	20	48	90·1	42	95·1	31	99·0
8	21	50	90·7	44	95·3	33	99·0
8	22	53	90·3	46	95·5	35	99·0
8	23	55	90·9	49	95·2	36	99·1
8	24	58	90·6	51	95·4	38	99·1
8	25	61	90·2	54	95·1	40	99·1
9	9	22	90·6	18	96·0	12	99·2
9	10	25	90·5	21	95·7	14	99·2
9	11	28	90·5	24	95·4	17	99·0
9	12	31	90·5	27	95·1	19	99·1
9	13	34	90·4	29	95·7	21	99·1
9	14	37	90·4	32	95·4	23	99·1
9	15	40	90·4	35	95·2	25	99·2
9	16	43	90·5	38	95·1	28	99·0
9	17	46	90·5	40	95·5	30	99·1

Table 18.5 (*continued*)

		Level of confidence					
Sample sizes (n_1, n_2)		90% (approx)		95% (approx)		99% (approx)	
Smaller	Larger	K	Exact level (%)	K	Exact level (%)	K	Exact level (%)
9	18	49	90·5	43	95·4	32	99·1
9	19	52	90·5	46	95·2	34	99·1
9	20	55	90·5	49	95·1	37	99·0
9	21	58	90·6	51	95·5	39	99·1
9	22	61	90·6	54	95·4	41	99·1
9	23	64	90·6	57	95·3	44	99·0
9	24	67	90·6	60	95·1	46	99·0
9	25	70	90·6	63	95·0	48	99·1
10	10	28	91·1	24	95·7	17	99·1
10	11	32	90·1	27	95·7	19	99·2
10	12	35	90·7	30	95·7	22	99·1
10	13	38	91·2	34	95·1	25	99·0
10	14	42	90·4	37	95·2	27	99·1
10	15	45	90·9	40	95·2	30	99·0
10	16	49	90·3	43	95·3	32	99·1
10	17	52	90·7	46	95·4	35	99·1
10	18	56	90·1	49	95·5	38	99·0
10	19	59	90·6	53	95·0	40	99·1
10	20	63	90·0	56	95·1	43	99·0
10	21	66	90·4	59	95·2	45	99·1
10	22	69	90·8	62	95·3	48	99·1
10	23	73	90·4	65	95·3	51	99·0
10	24	76	90·7	68	95·4	53	99·1
10	25	80	90·3	72	95·0	56	99·1
11	11	35	91·2	31	95·3	22	99·2
11	12	39	90·9	34	95·6	25	99·1
11	13	43	90·7	38	95·3	28	99·1
11	14	47	90·5	41	95·6	31	99·1
11	15	51	90·3	45	95·3	34	99·1
11	16	55	90·1	48	95·6	37	99·1
11	17	58	90·9	52	95·3	40	99·1
11	18	62	90·8	56	95·1	43	99·1
11	19	66	90·6	59	95·3	46	99·1
11	20	70	90·5	63	95·1	49	99·1
11	21	74	90·4	66	95·4	52	99·1
11	22	78	90·3	70	95·2	55	99·1
11	23	82	90·2	74	95·0	58	99·1
11	24	86	90·1	77	95·3	61	99·1
11	25	90	90·0	81	95·1	64	99·1
12	12	43	91·1	38	95·5	28	99·2
12	13	48	90·2	42	95·4	32	99·0
12	14	52	90·5	46	95·4	35	99·1
12	15	56	90·7	50	95·3	38	99·1
12	16	61	90·0	54	95·3	42	99·0
12	17	65	90·3	58	95·2	45	99·1

Table 18.5 (*continued*)

| Sample sizes (n_1, n_2) | | 90% (approx) | | 95% (approx) | | 99% (approx) | |
Smaller	Larger	K	Exact level (%)	K	Exact level (%)	K	Exact level (%)
12	18	69	90·5	62	95·2	48	99·1
12	19	73	90·7	66	95·2	52	99·0
12	20	78	90·1	70	95·2	55	99·1
12	21	82	90·4	74	95·2	59	99·0
12	22	86	90·6	78	95·2	62	99·0
12	23	91	90·1	82	95·1	65	99·1
12	24	95	90·3	86	95·1	69	99·0
12	25	99	90·5	90	95·1	72	99·1
13	13	52	90·9	46	95·6	35	99·1
13	14	57	90·6	51	95·2	39	99·1
13	15	62	90·2	55	95·4	43	99·0
13	16	66	90·8	60	95·0	46	99·1
13	17	71	90·6	64	95·2	50	99·1
13	18	76	90·3	68	95·4	54	99·0
13	19	81	90·1	73	95·1	58	99·0
13	20	85	90·6	77	95·2	61	99·1
13	21	90	90·4	81	95·4	65	99·1
13	22	95	90·2	86	95·1	69	99·0
13	23	99	90·7	90	95·3	73	99·0
13	24	104	90·5	95	95·1	76	99·1
13	25	109	90·3	99	95·2	80	99·1
14	14	62	90·6	56	95·0	43	99·1
14	15	67	90·7	60	95·4	47	99·1
14	16	72	90·7	65	95·3	51	99·1
14	17	78	90·0	70	95·2	55	99·1
14	18	83	90·1	75	95·1	59	99·1
14	19	88	90·2	79	95·4	64	99·0
14	20	93	90·3	84	95·3	68	99·0
14	21	98	90·4	89	95·2	72	99·0
14	22	103	90·5	94	95·1	76	99·0
14	23	108	90·6	99	95·1	80	99·1
14	24	114	90·0	103	95·3	84	99·1
14	25	119	90·2	108	95·3	88	99·1
15	15	73	90·2	65	95·5	52	99·0
15	16	78	90·7	71	95·1	56	99·1
15	17	84	90·3	76	95·1	61	99·0
15	18	89	90·7	81	95·2	65	99·1
15	19	95	90·4	86	95·3	70	99·0
15	20	101	90·1	91	95·4	74	99·1
15	21	106	90·4	97	95·1	79	99·0
15	22	112	90·2	102	95·1	83	99·1
15	23	117	90·5	107	95·2	88	99·0
15	24	123	90·3	112	95·3	92	99·1
15	25	129	90·0	118	95·0	97	99·0

Table 18.5 (*continued*)

Sample sizes (n_1, n_2)		Level of confidence					
		90% (approx)		95% (approx)		99% (approx)	
Smaller	Larger	K	Exact level (%)	K	Exact level (%)	K	Exact level (%)
16	16	84	90·6	76	95·3	61	99·0
16	17	90	90·6	82	95·1	66	99·0
16	18	96	90·5	87	95·4	71	99·0
16	19	102	90·5	93	95·2	75	99·1
16	20	108	90·5	99	95·1	80	99·1
16	21	114	90·5	104	95·3	85	99·1
16	22	120	90·5	110	95·2	90	99·1
16	23	126	90·5	116	95·0	95	99·1
16	24	132	90·5	121	95·2	100	99·1
16	25	138	90·5	127	95·1	105	99·0
17	17	97	90·1	88	95·1	71	99·1
17	18	103	90·4	94	95·1	76	99·1
17	19	110	90·0	100	95·1	82	99·0
17	20	116	90·3	106	95·2	87	99·0
17	21	122	90·5	112	95·2	92	99·1
17	22	129	90·2	118	95·2	97	99·1
17	23	135	90·5	124	95·2	103	99·0
17	24	142	90·2	130	95·2	108	99·0
17	25	148	90·4	136	95·2	113	99·1
18	18	110	90·3	100	95·3	82	99·0
18	19	117	90·2	107	95·1	88	99·0
18	20	124	90·1	113	95·2	93	99·1
18	21	131	90·0	120	95·1	99	99·0
18	22	137	90·5	126	95·2	105	99·0
18	23	144	90·4	133	95·0	110	99·1
18	24	151	90·4	139	95·2	116	99·0
18	25	158	90·3	146	95·0	122	99·0
19	19	124	90·4	114	95·0	94	99·0
19	20	131	90·5	120	95·3	100	99·0
19	21	139	90·1	127	95·3	106	99·0
19	22	146	90·3	134	95·2	112	99·0
19	23	153	90·4	141	95·2	118	99·0
19	24	161	90·1	148	95·2	124	99·0
19	25	168	90·2	155	95·1	130	99·1
20	20	139	90·4	128	95·1	106	99·1
20	21	147	90·2	135	95·2	113	99·0
20	22	155	90·1	142	95·3	119	99·0
20	23	162	90·4	150	95·1	126	99·0
20	24	170	90·3	157	95·2	132	99·0
20	25	178	90·2	164	95·3	139	99·0
21	21	155	90·3	143	95·1	119	99·1
21	22	163	90·4	151	95·0	126	99·1
21	23	171	90·4	158	95·2	133	99·1

Table 18.5 (*continued*)

Sample sizes (n_1, n_2)		90% (approx)		95% (approx)		99% (approx)	
			Exact		Exact		Exact
Smaller	Larger	K	level (%)	K	level (%)	K	level (%)
21	24	180	90·1	166	95·2	140	99·0
21	25	188	90·2	174	95·1	147	99·0
22	22	172	90·2	159	95·1	134	99·0
22	23	180	90·5	167	95·1	141	99·0
22	24	189	90·3	175	95·2	148	99·1
22	25	198	90·1	183	95·2	156	99·0
23	23	190	90·0	176	95·0	149	99·0
23	24	199	90·1	184	95·2	156	99·1
23	25	208	90·1	193	95·1	164	99·0
24	24	208	90·3	193	95·2	165	99·0
24	25	218	90·1	202	95·2	173	99·0
25	25	228	90·1	212	95·1	181	99·0

For samples sizes where n_1 and n_2 are greater than the range shown in the table, a satisfactory approximation to the value of K can be calculated as

$$K = \frac{n_1 n_2}{2} - \left(z_{1-\alpha/2} \times \sqrt{\frac{n_1 n_2 (n_1 + n_2 + 1)}{12}} \right),$$

rounded up to the next higher integer value, where $z_{1-\alpha/2}$ is the appropriate value from the standard Normal distribution for the $100(1 - \alpha/2)$ percentile.

For $n_1 = 25$, $n_2 = 10$, and $\alpha = 0.05$, for example, this calculation gives 71·3, which results in $K = 72$ for finding the 95% confidence interval, the same value as shown in the table.

For an explanation of the use of this table see chapter 5.

Table 18.6 Values of K^* for use in calculating confidence intervals for population medians in single samples or for differences between population medians for the case of two paired samples with sample size n from 6 to 50 and the associated exact levels of confidence, based on the Wilcoxon matched pairs signed rank sum distribution (see footnote overleaf)

Sample size (n)	Level of confidence					
	90% (approx)		95% (approx)		99% (approx)	
	K^*	Exact level (%)	K^*	Exact level (%)	K^*	Exact level (%)
6	3	90·6	1	96·9	—	—
7	4	92·2	3	95·3	—	—
8	6	92·2	4	96·1	1	99·2
9	9	90·2	6	96·1	2	99·2
10	11	91·6	9	95·1	4	99·0
11	14	91·7	11	95·8	6	99·0
12	18	90·8	14	95·8	8	99·1
13	22	90·6	18	95·2	10	99·2
14	26	90·9	22	95·1	13	99·1
15	31	90·5	26	95·2	16	99·2
16	36	90·7	30	95·6	20	99·1
17	42	90·2	35	95·5	24	99·1
18	48	90·1	41	95·2	28	99·1
19	54	90·4	47	95·1	33	99·1
20	61	90·3	53	95·2	38	99·1
21	68	90·4	59	95·4	43	99·1
22	76	90·2	66	95·4	49	99·1
23	84	90·2	74	95·2	55	99·1
24	92	90·5	82	95·1	62	99·0
25	101	90·4	90	95·2	69	99·0
26	111	90·1	99	95·1	76	99·1
27	120	90·5	108	95·1	84	99·0
28	131	90·1	117	95·2	92	99·0
29	141	90·4	127	95·2	101	99·0
30	152	90·4	138	95·0	110	99·0
31	164	90·2	148	95·2	119	99·0
32	176	90·2	160	95·0	129	99·0
33	188	90·3	171	95·2	139	99·0
34	201	90·2	183	95·2	149	99·0
35	214	90·3	196	95·1	160	99·0
36	228	90·2	209	95·0	172	99·0
37	242	90·2	222	95·1	183	99·0
38	257	90·1	236	95·1	195	99·0
39	272	90·1	250	95·1	208	99·0
40	287	90·3	265	95·0	221	99·0
41	303	90·2	280	95·0	234	99·0
42	320	90·1	295	95·1	248	99·0
43	337	90·0	311	95·1	262	99·0
44	354	90·1	328	95·0	277	99·0
45	372	90·0	344	95·1	292	99·0
46	390	90·1	362	95·0	308	99·0
47	408	90·2	379	95·1	323	99·0
48	427	90·2	397	95·1	340	99·0
49	447	90·1	416	95·1	356	99·0
50	467	90·1	435	95·1	374	99·0

For sample sizes of n over 50, a satisfactory approximation to the value of K^* can be calculated as

$$K^* = \frac{n(n+1)}{4} - \left(z_{1-\alpha/2} \times \sqrt{\frac{n(n+1)(2n+1)}{24}}\right),$$

rounded up to the next higher integer value, where $z_{1-\alpha/2}$ is the appropriate value from the standard Normal distribution for the $100(1-\alpha/2)$ percentile.

For $n = 50$ and $\alpha = 0.05$, for example, this calculation gives 434·5, which results in $K^* = 435$ for finding the 95% confidence interval, the same value as shown in the table.

For an explanation of the use of this table see chapter 5.

Index